Discourse Impairments

Discourse Impairments

Assessment and Intervention Applications

Lynn S. Bliss

University of Houston

Allyn and Bacon
Boston • London • Toronto • Sydney • Tokyo • Singapore

Editor in Chief, Education: Paul A. Smith
Executive Editor: Stephen D. Dragin
Editorial Assistant: Barbara Strickland
Marketing Manager: Kathleen Morgan
Editorial Production Administrator: Bryan Woodhouse
Editorial-Production Service: Chestnut Hill Enterprises, Inc.
Composition and Prepress Buyer: Linda Cox
Manufacturing Buyer: Chris Marson
Cover Administrator: Kristina Mose-Libon
Electronic Composition: Publisher's Design and Production Services, Inc.

Between the time Website information is gathered and then published, it is not unusual for some sites to have closed. Also, the transcription of URLs can result in unintended typographical errors. The publisher would appreciate notification where these occur so that they may be corrected in subsequent editions.

Library of Congress Cataloging-in-Publication Data

Bliss, Lynn S.
     Discourse impairments : assessment and intervention applications / Lynn S. Bliss.—1st ed.
        p.   cm.
     Includes bibliographical references and index.
     ISBN 0-205-33407-5
     1. Language disorders in children—Diagnosis.   2. Discourse analysis.   I. Title
     RJ496.L35B5485   2002
     618.92'855—dc21   2001046135

Printed in the United States of America

10 9 8 7 6 5 4 3 2 1   06 05 04 03 02 01

To the memory of Carol Ann Prutting, who has continued to inspire me throughout my professional career. Her memory has guided me to instill pragmatics throughout all of my professional thoughts. She is missed.

Contents

Part Five   Intervention   135

Part Six   Answers for Selected Chapters in Text
Chapters 2, 4, 6, 8, 10, 12, 14, 16, 18, 20, and 22   153

Answers in the Instructor's Manual

Chapters 3, 5, 7, 9, 11, 13, 15, 17, 19, 21

Preface

The impetus for *Discourse Impairments: Assessment and Intervention Applications* originated from my professional experiences with students and clinicians. Originally, my presentations consisted mostly of lectures. While my audiences gained knowledge of material that I presented, there was minimal direct application of the information that I described. I decided to change my approach to increase the clinical relevance and application of my material. I included discourse samples and exercises in the form of related questions that enabled my audience to apply to clinical contexts the information that I had presented. The result was that both students and clinicians increased their analytical and interpretive skills from completing the exercises. The unique feature of this book is the inclusion of discourse samples that serve as the basis for learning about childhood language disorders as well as their assessment and treatment.

The purpose of *Discourse Impairments: Assessment and Intervention Applications* is to facilitate critical thinking as it relates to the nature of childhood language disorders and their assessment and intervention. It is comprised of the following sections:

Part One: Identification of Critical Features of Language Behavior

In this section, the reader will learn to identify critical aspects of language behavior, including the analysis of early communicative functioning, semantic relations, syntactic categories, sentence structure, and discourse coherence. The purpose of this section is to provide the reader with information that is needed to analyze discourse samples from children at different levels of functioning. It does not represent a complete analysis; there are aspects of functioning that are omitted (e.g., word endings, irregular verb and noun forms, and phonological production). The features that are included reflect some of the most prominent aspects of childhood language disorders.

Part Two: Childhood Language Disorders

The purpose of this section is to enable readers to identify the primary characteristics of childhood language disorders and apply this knowledge to assessment and intervention of symptoms. The disorders that are discussed are specific language impairment, adolescent language learning disorders, mental retardation, hearing impairment, autism, and traumatic brain injury.

Part Three: Cultural and Linguistic Diversity

In this section, the reader will distinguish between African American dialect features and symptoms of a disorder and between features of limited English proficiency and symptoms of a disorder. Samples have been elicited from African American and Spanish-speaking children. Features of typical and impaired language development are contrasted.

Part Four: Assessment

Issues pertaining to assessment are presented, such as language variation as a function of different contexts (e.g., home and clinic elicitations) and discourse genres (e.g., conversation and narratives). In addition, the variability between results of standardized testing and discourse is explored. Finally, a comprehensive analysis of discourse is presented. All of the issues in this section need to be understood in order to make appropriate clinical decisions regarding a child's discourse abilities.

Part Five: Intervention

Intervention strategies are described for the remediation of some of the symptoms evident in childhood language disorders. An interactive, functional approach is described in which generalization of new behaviors is fostered using discourse in natural contexts.

Part Six: Selected Answers

Answers to some of the exercises are presented (the other answers are located in the *Instructor's Manual*). If you do not do each exercise, you should read the answers because additional information is presented in this section that pertains to some of the topics under discussion. The answers are only suggestions. Although the samples have been analyzed frequently and the questions answered often by many individuals, differences of opinion have occurred. The answers to some questions are based on clinical experience that will differ among clinicians. There will be other interpretations of the answers that will be valid. Let me know if you have questions or disagreements with my interpretations (lbliss@uh.edu). I enjoy discovering new interpretations of this material. Good luck!

Acknowledgments

A bouquet should be presented to all of my current and past students at Penn State University, Wayne State University, and the University of Houston, who collected many of the samples that have been included in this book. Flower arrangements are awarded to my professional colleagues in both Michigan and Texas. They contributed discourse samples and insights regarding the interpretation of the material. My colleague, Susann Dowling, should receive Texas roses; she was supportive of my endeavors and gave me valuable insights regarding the publishing process.

My consultants deserve trees planted in their honor. They identified my mistakes and gave me words of wisdom and guidance. Any errors in this book, however, are mine and not theirs. These wise people include Michael Clark, Western Michigan University; Linda M. Bland-Stewart, George Washington University; and Adelaida Restrepo, University of Georgia.

Corsages are presented to Martha K. Brennan, Saint Louis University, and Nickola Nelson, Western Michigan University, the reviewers who guided me and helped prune and weed the manuscript so that it would bloom. Finally, a green and white boutonniere goes to Steve Dragin for his counsel throughout my writing endeavors.

Discourse Impairments

1
Introduction

Discourse Impairments: Assessment and Intervention Applications was developed to foster an understanding of the nature of childhood language disorders and to enable readers to apply their knowledge to assessment and intervention. Discourse samples are presented that illustrate impairments frequently found in childhood language disorders. The framework for this book follows.

What is language? Language is a multifaceted, rule-governed system. It is comprised of diverse components and has been described from different, yet compatible, perspectives. The first approach focuses on the following interrelated dimensions of language: syntax (e.g., grammatical categories, words, and sentence structure), pragmatics (e.g., communicative intent and discourse), content (e.g., meaning of utterances), morphology (e.g., bound morphemes), and phonology (e.g., regularities of the sound system).

The second perspective reflects the model described by Bloom and Lahey (1978). Language is comprised of three interacting and interrelated dimensions: form, content, and use. Form represents the syntactic, morphological, and phonological aspects of language. Content reflects semantics, meaning relationships that are expressed and understood. Use refers to the pragmatic aspects of language. These categories are useful when describing language impairments to teachers and parents because they are easily understood by non–speech-language pathologists (Nelson, 1998).

Other related aspects of language are paralinguistics and nonlinguistic features that contribute to language. Paralinguistic features reflect prosody—changes in pitch and volume that enhance a message. For example, listeners distinguish between a sarcastic message and a sincere one based upon the prosodic elements of the message. Paralinguistic features help to contrast statements from some questions. Nonlinguistic features include facial expressions, gestures, and eye contact that serve to augment the meaning in a message.

Another parameter of language is modality, which encompasses comprehension and production. Modality reflects auditory comprehension, reading, speaking, and writing. These components are evident in the diverse aspects of language (e.g., syntax, semantics, form, content, and use).

What is discourse? Discourse reflects the pragmatic aspect of language. It refers to verbal interactions between two or more participants. The use of words is not always necessary to exchange information and have discourse. For example, users of sign language engage in discourse without the use of words. In this book, discourse refers to primarily verbal exchanges of information in communicative contexts.

I have used the term, "discourse," to reflect a broad category that can be applied to the study of most aspects of language. It influences how we speak, including our choice of grammatical categories, sentences, and concepts (Bates, 1976). The selection of pronouns, adjectives, articles, and specific sentence structures is influenced by a speaker's motivation to communicate and the perceived needs of the conversational participants. For example, a speaker will use an adjective to provide details and will use a particular sentence structure to highlight information.

There are several types of discourse, including conversation, narration (e.g., stories), and expository (e.g., formal and classroom interactions) exchanges. Conversational discourse was selected as the primary source for analysis in this book because it provides a realistic assessment of how a speaker uses words and sentences in naturalistic contexts (Paul, 2001). Most aspects of language can be evaluated with this type of sample.

What influences discourse? Discourse is influenced by context, which consists of participants, settings, and the motivations of conversational participants. Speakers modify their utterances when talking in informal and formal contexts, to known and unknown listeners, and to one or more individuals. Language is a social function and should be studied within an interpersonal context. Discourse also varies with cultural and linguistic backgrounds. Dialect use and bilingualism influence how we speak. These influences will affect the assessment of language behavior and our clinical judgments.

What is a language disorder? A language disorder is characterized by impairments in one or all of the dimensions and modalities that have been described. Language disorders reflect disruptions of syntax, pragmatics, semantics, morphology, and/or phonology. Language pathology can also be characterized by impairments in form, content, and use. Language disorders may be affected in the modalities of both comprehension and production or mainly in the production modality (Craig & Evans, 1993). Some children have primarily expressive impairments, while other children will manifest impaired comprehension and production.

Children with language disorders represent a diverse population. Individual differences are common with children of the same intelligence quotient or etiology. Clinicians should not expect every child to exhibit the same or all of the symptoms reflected in the samples included here.

How are language disorders described? In this book, two perspectives regarding the study of childhood language disorders are presented, although other approaches have also been described (Nelson, 1998; Paul, 2001). One approach focuses on the symptoms of childhood language pathology without consideration of etiology (Parts One, Four, and Five). This noncategorical approach enables clinicians to evaluate symptoms and behaviors. In the other approach, etiology is identified with respect to childhood language disorders (Part Two). The symptoms of specific language impairment, language learning disorders in adolescents, mental retardation, hearing loss, autism, and traumatic brain injury are described with respect to their primary symptoms. This approach is utilized in many school districts where there are special classes for children with different disabilities. However, recent efforts have been made to enable children with special needs to adapt to regular classrooms, following the guidelines of federal legislation, The Individuals with Disabilities Education Act of 1990 (IDEA).

How are language disorders identified? The assessment and identification of a language disorder is typically made on the basis of objective and subjective data (Allen, Bliss, & Timmons, 1981; Aram, Morris, & Hall, 1993). One type of information is derived from test data. Test scores that fall below the 10th percentile or 1.25 standard deviations below the mean would generally be considered to reflect a language disorder (Fey, 1986; Lee, 1974; Paul, 2001; Tomblin, Records, & Zhang, 1996).

The subjective process includes interpreting discourse, case history data, information from teachers and other sources, nonstandardized measures, and behavioral observations. The clinician determines whether the speaker's communication appears to be appropriate and reflects that of the child's peers. Test data and more subjective analyses are not always congruent (Allen, Bliss, & Timmons, 1981; Aram, Morris, & Hall, 1993). The skilled clinician weighs all of the evidence to identify a language impairment. Language assessment is both an art and a science (Allen, Bliss, & Timmons, 1981).

How is discourse assessed? Discourse samples are collected by conversing with a child about familiar topics, transcribing all of the utterances, and analyzing the sample with respect to different dimensions of language. These should be at least 50 utterances and they should be collected in different situations (Lund & Duchan, 1993). In this book the samples have been reduced to 20 to 50 utterances, a practice that is not suggested clinically. The samples were reduced to ease the task of analyzing the material. Clinicians should always attempt to elicit longer samples whenever possible. The focus here is on conversational discourse in contrast to other discourse genres, such as narratives and expository production. These genres can replace or supplement conversational samples.

One challenge in transcribing a sample is to identify specific utterances. Typically speakers combine their utterances and do not produce clear utterance boundaries. The challenge is to segment a sample into utterances that can be analyzed. There are a number of systems that have been used to segment utterances (Lund & Duchan, 1993; Nelson, 1998). For *Discourse Impairments*, utterances were identified by numbering separately phrases that began with a coordinating conjunction (e.g., *and, and then, so, because*, etc.) (Lund & Duchan, 1993; Nelson, 1998). The aim was to identify relatively short utterances that could be readily analyzed. Paralinguistic features of prosody and nonlinguistic feature of gestures were considered in the segmentation process. These features enabled the transcriber to determine whether an utterance was a question or statement or if objects or locations were referenced by gestures.

The field of childhood language disorders is exciting and challenging. Clinicians have the opportunity to help children to develop a wonderful gift, the ability to communicate. I wish you success on the fascinating journey that you are undertaking. Please note that the answers in Part Six are suggestions. You may have different interpretations, so please contact me with your ideas (lbliss@uh.edu).

Part One

Identification of Critical Features of Language Behavior

The purposes of this section are to describe different components of language and discourse behavior that are vulnerable in childhood language disorders and to enable readers to analyze children's use of these dimensions. The features that have been selected are relevant for children with a variety of disorders and different levels of language development. They encompass a range of abilities, including conversational participation, semantic relations, syntax, and discourse. After completing this section, the reader will be able to analyze many aspects of language and communicative functioning. As to choices made regarding what features should be included, I selected features that are most prominent in childhood language disorders, based on my clinical experience and related research.

2
Early Conversational Functioning

Children with typical language development have a wide range of communicative skills that they use to interact with adults and peers. Children with language impairments may be limited in their communicative abilities. The communicative acts described in this section represent a partial description of an individual's communicative repertoire. A complete list can be found in Fey (1986).

Asssertive conversational acts consist of spontaneous: (1) information requests (e.g., questions—*What that? Where doggie?*); (2) action requests (e.g., commands and directions—*Move it. Put ball.*); (3) comments (e.g., labels or descriptions of objects and events and events—*Ball up* [describing the location of the ball], *Have tummy ache*); and (4) statements (e.g., descriptions of cognitive states, feelings, desires, evaluations, rules, etc.—*Want that. Yukky. Hafta go now.*).

Responsive conversational acts consist of the following: (1) answers (e.g., answers to requests for information—Q: *What is that?* A: *Ball.*); (2) action responses (e.g., responses to requests for action—Adult: *Move the ball here.* Child: *I moved it.*), and (3) statement responses (e.g., utterances that acknowledge or agree with the prior statement and do not add information—*Yeah, Oh*).

The following four communicative profiles are derived from the relative frequencies of the above communication acts (Fey, 1986):

Active conversationalists initiate and respond frequently, with relatively high frequencies of both assertives and responsives. They show an interest in interacting with others even though they have severe syntactic or phonological impairments. Some children with language disorders have a broad range of communicative functions and would be considered to be active conversationalists (Rom & Bliss, 1981).

Passive conversationalists are strong in the responsiveness domain. They respond to requests and do not initiate interactions. They are weak in the assertive domain. Some children with language and mental impairments have been described as passive conversationalists (Fey & Leonard, 1983; MacDonald, 1985; Rosenberg, 1982).

Inactive communicators do not often initiate and respond; they are low in both assertiveness and responsiveness. Children who are severely unintelligible or who have severe expressive impairments may be inactive communicators because they talk minimally to unfamiliar individuals and peers, even though they may interact more with family members.

Verbal noncommunicators initiate a variety of utterances; they fail to respond appropriately to requests and statements (made either by themselves or others). They do not maintain a topic; they may be hyperverbal. Some children with hydrocephaly have been described as verbal noncommunicators because they talk a lot but do not respond appropriately (Bloom & Lahey, 1978).

Early conversational acts generally emerge in the following sequence: requesting actions and objects, comments, statements, requesting information and response to requests for information, (Chapman, 1981; Dore, 1975; Paul, 2001). Children with delays in language development generally exhibit the same range of communicative functions as do children with typical language development (Leonard, Camarata, Rowan, & Chapman, 1982; Rom & Bliss, 1981). However, some children may not use many comments and may use more responsives in comparison to their peers with typical language development (Leonard et al., 1982). Young children with hearing impairments and mental retardation have a full range of communicative functions (Curtiss, Prutting, & Lowell, 1979; Owens & MacDonald, 1982; Skarakis & Prutting, 1977). In contrast, children with autism exhibit different profiles of communicative functioning from children with typical language development. They tend to be limited in the social interactive functions of requesting, greeting, and acknowledging (Wetherby & Prutting, 1984).

Assessment Applications

1. Conversational samples that are longer than the one presented in this section are needed to obtain a comprehensive assessment of a child's communicative abilities.

2. Absence of a category does not mean that the child is unable to express himself or herself adequately. Elicitation procedures, the nonlinguistic context, and content of discourse influence the use of conversational acts. For example, a child may not need to express an assertive if there is no need to make a request. In order to study a wide range of communicative acts, tasks that are designed to elicit specific communicative behaviors may be useful (e.g., withholding a toy in order to elicit an assertive conversational act) (Bliss, 1993; Coggins, Olswang, & Guthrie, 1987; Owens, 1999; Wetherby, Cain, Yonclas, & Walker, 1988). In addition, a parent questionnaire or interview should be used as a means of determining the range of communicative acts that a child produces at home as well as in a clinical context.

3. Diversity of communicative acts and the words used to express them should be explored (Paul, 2001).

Intervention Applications

1. Clinicians should focus on increasing the frequency or range of communicative acts (e.g., questions, commands, answers) and increasing vocabulary (e.g., specific words) used to express these communicative acts.

2. Parents and siblings need to be an integral part of an intervention program. They should be taught how to elicit and respond to communicative attempts.

3. Clinicians should develop natural contexts (e.g., mealtime, bathing, play activities) as a means of eliciting a variety of communicative functions (Bliss, 1993).

Introduction to Sample

In this section the communicative functioning of Cameron, aged 3 ½ years, will be studied. He has been in a language intervention program for six months.

Cameron

3½ years

Adult: What do you want?

Cameron: 1. Want that [points to bubble bottle].

A: Do you wanna play with the bubbles? [nods yes] What are you doing?

C: 2. Opening [he opens a desk drawer].

A: Opening what?

C: 3. Brush [he finds a toothbrush].

A: What are you doing?

C: 4. Brush teeth [he begins to brush his teeth and then takes a pen out of the drawer].

A: Put the pen back.

C: 5. Want paper. 6. Paper on [sees paper on the clinician's desk].

A: Here's some paper.

C: 7. Bubble [points to a bottle of bubbles].

A: Look [clinician blows some bubbles]. Now it's your turn.

C: 8. More bubbles [he blows some bubbles].

A: Are you trying to eat the bubbles? [he tries to pop the bubbles with his mouth].

C: 9. Yuk. 10. Eat bubble [opens mouth and pretends to eat the bubbles] . . . . 11. Teeth. [he finds a set of teeth on top of the desk and shows them to the adult].

A: What are you doing?

C: 12. Up [throws a piece of paper in the air].

A: Yes, the paper went up. Now I'll throw it [the paper goes behind a toy box; he looks behind the toy box and tries to push the box to get the paper].

C: 13. Move it [Adult then moves the toy box away from the wall]. 14. Balloon [a red balloon is behind the toy box].

A: A balloon. Give me the balloon please.

C: 15. Blow it [hands the balloon to the adult who blows it up].

A: Do you want me to help you blow it?

C: 16. More.

A: There [clinician helps the child]. Do you want me to make it go up?

C: 17. More up.

A: It went up.

C: 18. Table on [the balloon lands on the table].

A: It's all over the room [they hit the balloon in different locations].

C: 19. There [he points to the balloon behind a chair]. 20. That? [points to a tape recorder] . . . . 21. Ryan? [a child who has therapy after Cameron].

A: Ryan's not here yet. Do you want me to blow the balloon up again?

C: 22. Up. 23. Up more [the balloon falls to the ground]. 24. Blow up.

A: OK, I'll blow more. Look at it now.

C: 25. Big.

A: Now it is big. Do you want me to tie the balloon?

C: 26. Tie it.

A: What are you doing? [Cameron climbs on a table and sits on it].

C: 27. Sit down. 28. Light off [an adult comes in and turns off the light in the room].

A: Yes, the light went off. Turn it back on [addressed to the adult].

C: 29. Light on. 30. OK.

Questions

1. Read Cameron's sample and identify each of Cameron's utterances in the categories presented below. Follow these guidelines:

   a. Some utterances are difficult to interpret. They can be classified in many ways, depending upon the context. You do not have a video of the child, so the task can be difficult. Look at the preceding or following utterance; the adult sometimes has interpreted the communicative function of an utterance, depending upon Cameron's behavior or nonlinguistic cues. Coding communicative acts is not an objective procedure. I will give you my rationales for coding specific utterances that may be difficult to interpret. You may have different interpretations. There will not always be correct answers.

   This is a difficult exercise because of the subjectivity of the analysis. Don't be discouraged!!

   b. The "other" category is used when an utterance does not fit any of the categories below. I have reduced the number of categories. There may be utterances that do not fit into this limited coding system.

Assertive Conversational Acts

Requests for information:

Requests for action:

Comments:

Statements:

Total number of assertives:

Responsive Conversational Acts

Answers:

Action responses:

Statement responses:

Total number of responses:

Other

Other:

Total number of other:

2. Based on your analysis, what type of communicator is Cameron? Support your answer.

3. Does Cameron need intervention to increase his repertoire of conversational acts? Support your answer.

4. List two intervention goals for the following conversational profiles.

Passive conversationalist:

Inactive communicator:

Verbal noncommunicator:

3
Semantic Relations

Semantic relations reflect meanings that a child expresses. In this section we will focus on two-word utterances because they are most often analyzed (Brown, 1972). The most frequent semantic relations are (Brown, 1973):

Agent + Action: *John hit*

Action + Object: *Eat cookie*

Agent + Object: *Mary juice*

Demonstrative + Entity: *This doll*

Attribute + Entity: *Big chair*

Entity + Locative: *book* [on the] *table*

Possessor + Possession: *Sue*['s]*doll*

Recurrence: *More milk*

Disappearance: *Allgone juice*

Negation: *No milk*

Other: *Light off*

These semantic relations are identified by context. For example, negation may signal one of three meanings, depending upon the speaker's intent and the situation (Bloom, 1973). In one context, *no milk* can represent the concept of nonexistence, in which milk was present but is no longer present. In another context, *no milk* means denial, as in *this is not milk; it is juice*. Finally, *no milk* could signal rejection, (e.g., I don't want milk; I want juice).

The "other" category represents utterances that cannot be scored by the categories specified above. According to Paul (2001), 30 percent of utterances in a language sample would be typically represented by this category. If this number is above 50 percent, an analysis of the types of meanings that have been encoded should be carried out. For some children, advanced meanings might be expressed, such as causality, as in *broke* [because it] *fell*; manner, *go quick*[ly] or time *went today* (Paul, 2001). A child with delayed expressive development who conveyed these meanings would exhibit advanced cognitive growth. Particle expressions also consist of the "other" category, such as *sit down* and *light off*.

The earliest semantic relations that emerge are negation and recurrence (Bloom, 1973; Bloom, Lightbown, & Hood, 1975; Brown, 1973). Agents, actions, and objects take prominence by the time a child is three years old (Bloom, 1973; Brown, 1972). They are the basis for adult sentence structure and need to be expressed by all children.

There is variability in the use of semantic relations by children with language disorders. Most children with specific language impairment, hearing impairment, and mental retardation express a broad range of semantic relations, similar to the repertoire found in the utterances of children with typical language development (Coggins, 1979; Freedman & Carpenter, 1976; Leonard, Bolders, & Miller, 1976; Morehead & Ingram, 1973; Skarakis & Prutting, 1977). However, some children with language disorders do not produce many agents or agent + action + object structures (Lee, 1966; Leonard, 1972). These patterns suggest that a child does not have the basis for adult sentence structure (e.g., agent + action + object or subject + verb + object forms). They may use particles rather than agent + action forms (Leonard, 1972). Children with language disorders do not represent a homogeneous group; their language behavior needs to be studied for their individual differences.

Assessment Applications

1. Normative data that describe the relative frequencies of the use of semantic relations are not available. They are difficult to obtain because the use of semantic relations is contextually based. For example, if the topic of possession did not occur in a language sample elicitation, a child would not be expected to use this semantic relation. Absence of a concept does not mean

that the child does not understand or use a concept. Additional sampling, parent interviews, and eliciting specific semantic relations are needed to enable a clinician to obtain a thorough assessment of a child's abilities.

2. A semantic analysis will provide clinicians with important information regarding the flexibility in using different semantic relations. Clinicians need to determine if a child is limited to using mainly the relations of recurrence, location, and objects or entities and does not use many agents and actions. This pattern would show inflexibility in the range of semantic relations. However, before age three, children may show a preference for specific semantic relations (Lahey, 1988).

3. The clinician also needs to examine the words used to express semantic relations. For example, a child may be limited to using only *I* and *mommy* to express agents (Lee, 1966). This child would have a limited lexical repertoire.

Intervention Applications

1. Meaningful contexts (e.g., eating, dressing) should be established in which a variety of semantic relations are focused and are given opportunities for expression (Bliss, 1993). Semantic relations should be modeled in play contexts.

2. Concepts such as recurrence and negation should receive early focus for children with severe language impairments (Bliss, 1993).

3. Flexibility can be enhanced by either increasing vocabulary in existing semantic relations (e.g., *Mommy cook, daddy cook, John cook*) or increasing the variety of semantic relations (e.g., agent + action, possessor + possession), depending upon the abilities of a child.

Cameron

3½ years

Adult: What do you want?

Cameron: 1. Want that [points to bubble bottle].

A: Do you wanna play with the bubbles? [nods yes] What are you doing?

C: 2. Opening [he opens a desk drawer].

A: Opening what?

C: 3. Brush [he finds a toothbrush].

A: What are you doing?

C: 4. Brush teeth [he begins to brush his teeth and then takes a pen out of the drawer].

A: Put the pen back.

C: 5. Want paper. 6. Paper on [sees paper on the clinician's desk].

A: Here's some paper.

C: 7. Bubble [points to a bottle of bubbles].

A: Look [clinician blows some bubbles]. Now it's your turn.

C: 8. More bubbles [he blows some bubbles].

A: Are you trying to eat the bubbles? [he tries to pop the bubbles with his mouth].

C: 9. Yuk. 10. Eat bubble [opens mouth and pretends to eat the bubbles] . . . . . 11. Teeth [he finds a set of teeth on top of the desk and shows them to the adult].

A: What are you doing?

C: 12. Up [throws a piece of paper in the air].

A: Yes, the paper went up. Now I'll throw it [the paper goes behind a toy box; he looks behind the toy box and tries to push the box to get the paper].

C: 13. Move it [Adult then moves the toy box away from the wall]. 14. Balloon [a red balloon was behind the toy box].

A: A balloon. Give me the balloon please.

C: 15. Blow it [hands the balloon to the adult who blows it up].

A: Do you want me to help you blow it?

C: 16. More.

A: There [clinician helps the child]. Do you want me to make it go up?

C: 17. More up.

A: It went up.

C: 18. Table on [the balloon land on the table].

A: It's all over the room [they hit the balloon in different locations].

C: 19. There [he points to the balloon behind a chair]. 20. That? [points to a tape recorder] . . . . . 21. Ryan? [a child who has therapy after Cameron].

A: Ryan's not here yet. Do you want me to blow the balloon up again?

C: 22. Up. 23. Up more [the balloon falls to the ground]. 24. Blow up.

A: OK, I'll blow more. Look at it now.

C: 25. Big.

A: Now it is big. Do you want me to tie the balloon?

C: 26. Tie it.

A: What are you doing? [Cameron climbs on a table and sits on it].

C: 27. Sit down. 28. Light off [an adult comes in and turns off the light in the room].

A: Yes, the light went off. Turn it back on [addressed to the adult].

C: 29. Light on. 30. OK.

Questions

1. List Cameron's two-word utterances (I found 16).

1.   9.

2.   10.

3.   11.

4.   12.

5.   13.

6.   14.

7.   15.

8.   16.

2. Identify the agent + action, action + object and agent + object structures.

3. Does Cameron exhibit the basis of adult sentence structure? Support your answer.

4. Does Cameron express the concepts of recurrence, negation, possession, and attribution in his two-word utterances? If so, where? Does Cameron use particles? If so, where?

5. What would be your go als in therapy? Why?

6. Compare Cameron's pragmatic and semantic abilities. Which are stronger? Why?

4
Verb and Noun Phrase Expansion

One indicator of language development is the expansion of the verb and noun phrase. The verb phrase consists of the main verb, auxiliary system, adverbs, and prepositions with optional phrases (James, 1990; McLauglin, 1998; Retherford, 1993). The copula and auxiliary verbs are vulnerable in language pathology (Bliss, 1989; Conti-Ramsden & Jones, 1997; Hadley, 1998a; Rice, 1994). The noun phrase includes modifiers before the noun, such as articles, possessives, and demonstratives.

Verb Phrase

Copula verbs:

> Forms of *be* + noun, adverb or adjective
> Examples: *I'm mad.*
> *John was fast.*
> *They were pretty.*

Auxiliary verbs:

> Forms of *be* + verb + *ing*
> Examples: *Jane's swimming.*
> *Was she running?*
> *They were leaving.*

There are auxiliary forms; they are not as relevant to early language development because they represent advanced linguistic functioning (e.g., perfective, HAVE + verb + optional inflection).

Modal auxiliary verbs:

> *can, could; will, would; may, might, must; shall, should*

They represent the following meanings: ability/inability/permission (*can/can't*), intention/ nonintention (*should/shouldn't*), possibility/probability (*may, might*), and conditionality (*could/couldn't*).

Do as an auxiliary verb:

> Examples: *Did he go?*
> *She didn't leave.*
> *They did see me!*
> *How does it work?*

Most of these forms can occur as contractible or contractible forms.

> *Contractible* forms: '*m* (*am*), '*s* (*is*), '*re* (*are*), '*d* (*would*) and '*ll* (*will*)

> I'*m* mad; She'*s* busy; They'*re* tired; I'*ll* leave.

Uncontractible forms:

> *was, were, can, could, shall, should,* and *do*
> *is, are, would,* and *will* in the following contexts:
>   utterance initial position
> *Is he sick? Is she crying? Will they leave?*
>   utterance final position
> *Yes, he is.*
>   utterances produced with emphasis
> *She is here!*

Note that am/'m, is/'s and are/'re can be either contractible or uncontractible. The usage depends upon the linguistic context. Uncontractible forms generally occur in the initial and final position of utterances and with emphasis.

The uncontractible copula and auxiliary emerge before the contractible copula auxiliary (Brown, 1973). *Can* and *will* develop before *should* and *could*. *May, might,* and *must* are learned last (Bliss, 1989). Verbs and auxiliaries are more vulnerable than nouns in language pathology (Rice & Wexler, 1996; Watkins, 1994). Auxiliary verbs are more often deleted than copulas (Bliss, 1989; Ingram, 1972). Contractible forms tend to be omitted more than uncontractible forms (Bliss, 1989; Ingram, 1974).

Assessment Applications

1. Copula and auxiliary productions vary with dialect usage. For example, in African American English, these forms are not always present (Washington & Craig, 1994). Their absence does not indicate a language disorder (see Chapter 13).

2. Word endings (e.g., inflections) should also be assessed. Noun word endings (e.g., plural and possessive *s*) may be more frequently produced than verb endings (e.g., third-person singular *s* and past *ed*) by children with specific language impairment (Rice, 1994).

3. Expect more copula verbs than auxiliary forms to be produced by children with language impairments (Hadley & Rice, 1996).

Intervention Applications

1. The verb system should receive early focus because of its vulnerability (Watkins, 1994).

2. Salient and meaningful forms should be elicited initially. The modals, *can* and *can't*, are appropriate targets after a child produces agent + action + object structures (Bliss, 1988; 1993).

3. Inflections should be relegated to the final stages of intervention because they are generally redundant. Past tense should be elicited before third-person singular forms (Rice, 1994).

Noun Phrase

Noun phrase elaboration consists of words that modify or precede a noun. Some elements of the noun phrase are (McLaughlin, 1998; Owens, 1996; Retherford, 1993):

Articles: *a, an, the*

Quantifiers and numbers: *some, all, both, each, one, three*

Possessives: *my, your, Mary's*

Demonstratives: *this, that, those, these*

Adjectives: *red, small, happy*

Demonstratives are early-acquired forms. Adjectives are used after a noun before preceding one. Multiple noun modifiers are rare until school age (Brown & Bellugi, 1964; McLauglin, 1998; Owens, 1996; Wells, 1985). Some common impairments in noun phrase development are the deletion of articles and absence or limited use of noun modifiers, reflecting a lack of elaboration of utterances (Bliss, 1989; Leonard, 1972).

Assessment Applications

1. Noun modifiers precede a noun in order to be considered part of the noun phrase. Noun modifiers are found only in utterances b, d, and f.

   a. *I saw <u>one</u>.*   **d.** *I have a <u>neat</u> room.*
   b. *I saw <u>one</u> book.*   **e.** *<u>That's</u> a car.*
   c. *It's <u>neat</u>.*   **f.** *I own <u>that</u> car.*

2. Clinicians should assess the types of errors children make. Most errors with the noun phrase occur as omissions of words, especially articles (Leonard, 1995). Redundant forms (e.g., *I bought <u>the a</u> toy*) are rare.

3. Use of the plural and possessive noun inflections should also be assessed and compared with the production of verb word endings.

Intervention Applications

1. Focus should be on grammatical categories that are perceptually salient, such as adjectives and quantifiers, and demonstratives in contrast to articles and noun inflections (Bliss, 1993).

2. Adjectives, quantifiers, and demonstratives should be elicited in contexts in which they are critical to communicate new information. For example, contrasting the words, *more* and *less* in a context of different amounts of juice highlight the concept of quantification. (Elicitation procedures for adjectives are presented in Chapter 20.)

3. If inflections are introduced, noun endings should be elicited before verb forms (Rice, 1994). Plural inflections are more amenable to treatment than are verb endings (Rice, 1994).

Introduction to Sample

Craig is 4 years, 10 months old. He has been enrolled in a university language intervention program for 6 months. He is delayed in language development.

Craig

4 years, 10 months

A: I'm just gonna turn the tape recorder on.

C: 1. No, want it off.

A: Why do you want it off?

C: 2. Because me no working. 3. It stay up here? [points to the tape recorder]

A: Yes. Let's play with this hospital set. What is this? [hospital bed]

C: 4. That's hospital bed.

A: What do you see? [toy object of a patient in the bed]

C: 5. Him hurting [the patient has a cast on his leg]. Uhoh!

A: What happened?

C: 6. It broken [points to the patient's leg]. 7. Hurt him leg. 8. Fix it.

A: It's broken.

C: 9. Can't fix it.

A: Who else do you see?

C: 10. Him doctor [points to a toy doctor]. 11. That needle [doctor had a needle]. 12. That thing shoe [points to the shoe of the patient]. 13. What this? [miniature sheet on the hospital bed covering the patient]

A: It's a sheet.

C: 14. Off [took off sheet]. 15. That off now. 16. This fall off [sheet]. 17. That off. Uhoh!

A: What's the matter?

C: 18. Him hands up [puts the patient's hands up]. 19. Him hand up.

A: Here's a dump truck [shows Craig a box with toys and takes the truck out of the box].

C: 20. That truck [points to the truck]. 21. It big. 22. Where's Shari? [his teacher] 23. What this? [holding a toy TV set]. 24. What this thing? 25. What this? 26. Something in here? [TV]. 27. Open this. 28. How you open this? [TV]

A: You don't open it. It's a TV.

C: 29. What her doing? [picture of a girl reading on the TV set]

A: She's reading.

Questions

1. Identify the utterances in which there is presence or absence of the copula, auxiliary, modal, and auxiliary *do/does*. Hint: Go through the sample and look for each feature separately. This way you won't miss anything.

copula verb present:

copula verb absent:

auxiliary verb present:

auxiliary verb absent:

modal auxiliary present:

modal auxiliary absent:

auxiliary *do/does* present:

auxiliary *do/does* absent:

2. A learned form is a series of words in a phrase or sentence that appear to be learned as a whole. It is also called an "unanalyzable chunk" because a child has not learned the words or segments independently. For example, a young child may say *What's that?* And not have mastered the copula verb because the *'s* and/or *is* are not used anywhere in the sample. Why might Craig's usage of *where's* and *that's* be learned forms?

3. Identify utterances characterized by either the presence or absence of articles, adjectives, and possessives and demonstratives before the noun.

Hints

    a. Even though a pronoun is used ungrammatically, it still counts as a noun modifier.

    b. A demonstrative must precede a noun for it to be considered a noun modifier.

Article + noun:

Absence of article:

Adjective + noun:

Possessive + noun:

Demonstrative + noun:

4. Perceptual saliency may influence the language production of children with language disorders. In this sample, compare Craig's use of articles versus demonstratives. How might perceptual saliency affect his performance?

5. What would be your goals for intervention for Craig? Why?

5
Complex Sentences

Analysis of complex sentences enables clinicians to assess the growth of later language development after sentences and basic noun and verb phrase elaboration have emerged. Sentences with two main verbs generally indicate a complex sentence, but there are some exceptions. Semiauxiliaries or introducers (e.g., *lemme, gonna, hafta, liketa, suposeda, hadta*) do not count as main verbs (Paul, 1981). They are semiauxiliaries (Paul, 1981). In some conjoined sentences a verb may be missing because it is optional and is understood (e.g., *Bill ate peas and Tara, corn*). Also, verbs derived from adjectives do not count as complex sentences (e.g., *We found a* <u>broken</u> *toy*). There are two types of complex sentences, conjoined and embedded.

Conjoined Sentences

In conjoined sentences, two clauses or sentences are linked by a conjunction.

Some *coordinating conjunctions* join two independent or main clauses (Hubbell, 1988). Coordinating conjunctions are *and, but, and then,* and *or*.

Subordinating conjunctions connect a main and secondary clause (Hubbell, 1988). Examples are: *because, if, so, unless,* and *when*.

Embedded Sentences

In embedded sentences a clause or sentence is included in another sentence (Craig & Washington, 1994; Nelson, 1988; Paul, 1981; Stefanni & Olson, 1998):

Infinitive complements are represented by the structure "verb/adjective-*to*-verb," as in

> I *promised to leave.* She *wanted to stay.* I'm *ready to eat.*

There are two types of infinitival complements:

Simple (<u>same subject</u>):

John <u>wanted to leave</u> (meaning John wanted himself to leave).

I <u>forgot to do</u> *my homework.*

Complex (different subject):

John wanted Bill to leave (meaning that Bill should leave).

Sue told <u>Steve to drive</u>.

Unmarked infinitives are utterances that have an infinitive without the *to* marker. Usually the words *make, help, watch,* or *let* are used.

> I <u>helped</u> [to] <u>cook</u> the dinner.
>
> <u>Let</u> me [to] <u>go</u> home early.

***That*-complements** are signaled by words of cognition, such as *guess, wish, hope, said, know, like* and *show*. The word *that* does not have to appear in this structure.

> I hope [that] <u>you will understand this sentence</u>.
>
> I wish [that] <u>you were able to complete this exercise</u>.

Simple noninfinitive *wh*-clauses occur when *who, what, where, when, why,* or *how* are present and the infinitival *to* marker is absent.

> I told you <u>what we did</u>.
>
> I know <u>where you went</u>.

***Wh*-infinitive clauses** occur when a *wh*-word (e.g., *what, where, who, how,* or *when*) and the infinitival *to* marker are present.

> Jacob knows <u>how to play soccer</u>.
>
> Marie forgot <u>where to park her car</u>.

Relative clauses are utterances in which a noun (or pronoun) is modified by a second clause. It may be preceded by *who, which* or *that*.

> *I like the girl <u>who is pretty</u>.*
> *I bought the book* [that] <u>*you liked.*</u>

Embedded and conjoined structures contain both an embedded and conjoined clause.

> *John <u>needs to study</u> when <u>Mary leaves</u>.*
> *She <u>likes to cook</u> because <u>it is fun</u>.*

Multiple embeddings occur when more than one embedded clause is present.

> *Sam <u>promised to tell</u> Jessy that <u>he would come to the party</u>.*
> *She <u>knows</u> that <u>they have to leave tomorrow</u>.*

Gerunds and participles are nouns formed from verbs (with an *ing* ending) or adjectives formed from verbs. They do not follow an auxiliary verb.

> *I like <u>shopping</u>* (gerund).
> *I saw the girl <u>hopping</u> around* (participle).

Early complex sentences, those generally mastered before four years, are: infinitive complements with the same subject, *that*-complements, simple *wh*-clauses, conjoined sentences, conjoined and embedded structures and multiple embeddings (Paul, 1981; 2001) Later structures, those that emerge after four years, are: infinitive complements with different subjects, relative clauses, *wh*-infinitives, unmarked infinitives, and gerunds and participles (Paul, 1981, 2001)

Children with language disorders may have difficulty in constructing complex sentences (Menyuk, 1964; Morehead & Ingram, 1973). Children with severe language disorders may not use them; their grammatical repertoire may be limited to phrases and simple sentences. Some children with milder language impairments have a similar repertoire of complex sentences to that of their peers with typical language development (Leonard, 1972; Morehead & Ingram, 1973). However, they produce more ungrammatical structures. The grammatical errors that frequently accompany complex sentences are: deletion of *to* in infinitival complements (e.g., *I need go*), non-agreement of tense in conjoined sentences (e.g., *Yesterday Bill <u>walked</u> and <u>will</u> fall*), omission or substitution of relative pronouns (e.g., *I saw Jane that* (for *who*) *was*

mad), and violation of word order in embedded clauses (e.g., *I know where is she*) (Johnston & Kamhi, 1984; Menyuk, 1964).

Assessment Applications

1. In a 50-utterance language sample, produced by a five-year-old child with typical language development, approximately 20 percent will be complex sentences (Paul, 1981).

2. Identification and segmentation of utterances is important when transcribing a language sample to identify complex sentences. Frequently children run their sentences together with multiple uses of *and* and *and then*. The system used in this chapter is one of a variety of approaches used to segment continuous discourse (see Lund Duchan, 1993, and Nelson, 1998, for a review of other approaches).

3. Absence of a type of complex sentence does not indicate an inability to produce the form. A child may not have had a communicative need to produce a structure in a discourse sample. The clinician will need to elicit additional forms.

Intervention Applications

1. Use of conversational recasts increases the frequency of complex sentences (Camarata, Nelson, & Camarata, 1994; Nelson, Camarata, Welsh, Butkovsky, & Camarata, 1996). In this procedure an adult uses a complex sentence after a child has produced a simple sentence. The adult's complex sentence should be semantically contingent to the child's utterance. It serves as a model for the child (e.g., if the child said, *I want, pen I want write;* the adult would respond, *You want to write with the pen*).

2. A child needs to know the concept of a conjunction before it is elicited. For example, a child needs to know the concept of causality before the conjunction *because* is elicited.

3. The conjunction *and* represents a variety of meanings and should be elicited in the following developmental order: additive (e.g., *a sock and a shoe*), temporal (e.g., *I got thirsty and got a glass and poured milk*), and causal (e.g., *I rode my bike too fast and I fell down*) (Bloom, Lahey, Hood, Lifter, & Feiss, 1980).

John

6 years, 3 months

J: 1. Lemme look at this [tape recorder].

A: No, because if you do, it will stop working.

J: 2. But where's it go? [looking at the tape moving]

A: The tape stays in the machine. Look in here [shows a bottle of bubbles].

J: 3. Lemme see what this is. 4. This bubbles! 5. Wanna blow some bubbles.

A: OK.

J: 6. Wanna blow some lots . . . 7. Do you how to open this? [bottle of bubbles]

A: Yes. Can you blow bubbles by yourself?

J: 8. Yeah, look what me doing [blows bubbles].

A: That was a lot of bubbles.

J: 9. Mamma gave me one of this before.

A: She did?

J: 10. Yeah, we gets money to get some. 11. Me gonna blow 'em way up here [gestures up]. 12. It hard to close it [tries to close the bottle].

A: You have to twist it. Do you wanna see what else is in the toy box?

J: 13. Me got boyfriend.

A: You do?

J: 14. Yeah, wanna know what name is?

A: What's his name?

J: 15. Matthew. 16. We play sand box by, by my alley.

A: Oh that's nice. How did you get your owie? [scratch on his face].

J: 17. Me falled.

A: Were you playing with your friend?

J: 18. Yeah, me . . . me . . . me . . . me got in. 19. Me try to climb up tree. 20. Me gonna pick some some apples and me fall down.

A: Oh, were there apples in the tree?

J: 21. Yeah, me try get 'em . . . . . 22. Matthew helped me.

A: I'm glad you didn't get hurt any worse. Here are some beads. You can put them on this string.

J: 23. Why don't me try this end? [tries to put bead where the knot is].

A: That end has a knot so the beads won't fall off.

J: 24. I gonna tie this double knot, OK? 25. You gonna teach to me how do it? 26. You know how to tie?

A: You know how to tie very well, don't you? Which bead would you like?

J: 27 . I hafta stick all my hand in there [where the beads are]. 28. Me try to figure out something. 29. Me gonna make my teachers makes.

A: OK.

J: 30. My moma got one this things [bead necklace]. 31. Me want you to help [string the beads].

A: OK.

J: 32. Me know how do with them. 33. You ready to try it? 34. I hope one of them on it [the string].

Questions

1. Identify all of the complex sentences (I found 17) and each type. If a complex structure is present in a sentence that contains grammatical errors, it should be considered a complex sentence (e.g., *Him need to go* should be considered to be an infinitive complement).

Utterance #	*Utterance*	*Type of Complex Sentence*
1.		
2.		
3.		
4.		
5.		
6.		
7.		
8.		
9.		
10.		
11.		
12.		
13.		
14.		
15.		
16.		
17.		

2. Does John have both earlier and later complex sentences? Support your answer.

3. John's complete language sample shows a mean length of utterance (MLU) of 5.59. At this stage of his language development (and at his chronological age), we would expect him to have mastered a variety of grammatical categories. However, he has difficulty with some of them. What grammatical categories are difficult for John?

4. What would be your goals for intervention for John?

5. Make up examples of three short complex sentences (different constructions) and one longer simple sentence. What do these differences suggest about using MLU as an index of language development above 5 years of age or above a MLU of 5.0?

6
Discourse Coherence

Discourse coherence refers to the clarity of a message, how clearly it is produced and understood. Speakers want to be understood and try to construct coherent messages. Sometimes individuals with typical language development are not always coherent; listeners cannot understand what they are attempting to say. For example, I once was reading a report and said to someone (who did not have access to the report), *I think she is a super candidate for admission.* My listener did not know the identity of the person in my utterance. This is an example of an error of discourse coherence. Children and adults with language disorders frequently produce messages that are not understood by a listener. Clinicians need to be able to describe the discourse coherence of children with language disorders.

Discourse coherence encompasses a variety of dimensions (Bliss, McCabe, & Miranda, 1998; Peterson & McCabe, 1983). Discourse coherence is expected because speakers and listeners have internalized a set of conversational principles (Grice, 1975). According to Grice (1975), conversational partners follow a set of implicit conversational rules that are designed to impart meaning. If any of the rules are not followed, discourse coherence is not achieved. The four conversational principles are (Grice, 1975):

1. Quantity: Provide a sufficient but not excessive amount of information to a listener.
2. Quality: Be truthful (we will assume this principle to be followed in the samples in this book because we do not have external evidence to verify the veracity of the children's utterances, unless otherwise noted).
3. Relation: Make your utterances relevant to a conversation.
4. Manner: Have your message organized, clear, and concise.

These rules can be used to study discourse coherence. In this chapter the focus will be on the whether a speaker maintains a topic of a conversation (relation), provides sufficient information for the listener to understand a message (quantity), identifies individuals who have been discussed (quantity), and produces a fluent message (manner). With inappropriate application of these conversational rules, a listener will not be able to easily understand what a speaker intends to communicate (Damico, 1985).

The dimensions of discourse coherence are:

Topic maintenance (relation) refers to how well utterances relate to each other or to a general topic. Reductions in topic maintenance result in discourse content that is rambling, associative, or tangential.

Informativeness (quantity) reflects the amount of information that a speaker provides to a listener. If information is omitted, a listener may not be able to understand what is conveyed and will need to infer the intended meaning. In narratives, young children and those with language disorders frequently omit information about the location of events and internal states, such as motivations, feelings, and reactions (Johnston, 1982; Miranda, McCabe & Bliss, 1998).

Referencing (quantity) refers to the identification of individuals, features and events (Bliss, McCabe, & Miranda, 1998; Miranda, McCabe & Bliss, 1998). The categories included under referencing function as cohesive devices—words that connect utterances (Halliday & Hassan, 1976). The following two types of referencing are the most frequent in the language samples that I have analyzed (for a complete discussion, see Halliday & Hassan, 1976):

Personal referencing requires that a pronoun or proper name be used after a referent has been identified. If a speaker said, *He is going*, the listener should be able to identify the referent for *he*. Similarly, a speaker needs to know who the individual is in the utterance, *Janey drove a new car.*

Lexical referencing indicates vocabulary specificity. For example, if a speaker said, *Maria did the fence*, the listener should be able to understand the meaning of the word *did* from a prior identification or context.

Did Maria fix or paint the fence? Inappropriate referencing occurs when general words are used that do not convey a specific meaning. Examples are: *stuff, something,* and *do.*

Fluency (manner) does not always affect the content of a message. It involves the smooth manner of production, how a speaker produces a message. It is related to discourse coherence because it affects the way participants understand a message. The dysfluencies that are discussed in this chapter are different from those evident in stuttering. In language use, word or phrase disruptions occur without extraneous facial movements or avoidance behaviors typically associated with stuttering. Dysfluencies cause the listener to make a special effort to understand a message. The most frequent types of dysfluencies are presented below (German, 1987, 1989; German & Simon, 1991; Peterson & McCabe, 1983):

Abandoned utterances: Utterances that are not completed, as in, *My mom has to . . . .*

Internal corrections: Retracings of words or phrases with corrections, as in, *We went in the water, went to the lake, uh beach, by up north.*

Repetitions: Word or phrasal reiterations that are not used for emphasis, as in, *I swim and and I I go home.*

Pauses: Long latencies between words, phrases, and/or utterances, as in, *I went . . . . to . . . . the zoo.*

Fillers: Use of *uh, er, like,* and other sounds or words that fill in an utterance, as in, *I um um um went with my brother um um to see um my dad um um who um um was in the hospital.* Caution should be exercised because all speakers use some fillers. Excessive use of fillers will interrupt the flow of conversation and may cause a listener to be distracted. Teenagers use *like* frequently; however, this filler generally does not disrupt discourse coherence.

Preschool children generally are able to produce coherent messages (Berman & Slobin, 1994; Peterson & McCabe, 1983). They maintain topic, provide sufficient information, and produce mostly fluent production (Ito, 1986; Peterson & McCabe, 1983). Children with language disorders exhibit impaired conversational abilities in all of the above dimensions (Biddle, McCabe, & Bliss, 1996; Liles, 1993; Miranda, McCabe, & Bliss, 1998). Coherence may vary with discourse task, conversation tends to be more coherent than narration (MacLachlan & Chapman, 1988).

Assessment Applications

1. Clinicians need to assess discourse coherence in a variety of types of messages; it will vary with length and type of discourse genre. Longer passages may be more reduced in coherence than shorter ones (Purcell & Liles, 1992). Conversational discourse is more coherent than narrative discourse (MacLachlan & Chapman, 1988).

2. I have used the following subjective categories to evaluate each discourse dimension.

   Appropriate: A dimension is appropriately used in the majority of utterances.

   Inappropriate: A dimension is used inappropriately in most of the utterances.

   Variable: A dimension varies in usage. This category is most common with the majority of children with language disorders.

3. Clinicians can establish a profile of overall discourse coherence by comparing a child's abilities and limitations among each dimension. This profile can be used to target specific features of discourse coherence.

Intervention Applications

1. Initial focus should be on the more general aspects of discourse coherence that influence an entire message, such as topic maintenance and informativeness. More specific aspects of discourse coherence should be targeted later, such as referencing and fluency.

2. Hierarchies should be implemented to increase discourse coherence. Shorter responses to questions should be elicited before ones that require elaboration; conversation should be targeted before narratives.

3. Topic maintenance deviations may indicate comprehension or attention deficits. These impairments will also need to be targeted in intervention.

Introduction to the Sample

In the sample in this section, Michael is conversing with his clinician. He is an African American male who is enrolled in a regular classroom. He has been enrolled in a language remediation program for two years.

Michael

8 years

Clinician: What do you do after school? Do you watch cartoons?

Michael: 1. Yep, at yesterday night I saw Halloween cartoon like something nasty from this witch. 2. She stick her thumb in her hand. 3. She go like this (gestures) 4. and some flowers be growing up.

C: What else happened in the cartoon?

M: 5. At the end, the, one those owls say "the pumpkin pie" 6. and when they say "pumpkin pie," the . . . 7. and the pumpkin say, "pumpkin pie?" 8. and the pumpkin be running.

C: When do you have pumpkin pie?

M: 9. Well, before at my house I eat pumpkin pie.

C: When do you have it?

M: 10. From last Halloween, something nasty be coming from pumpkin seeds.

C: Do you eat pumpkin seeds?

M: 11. No, it taste kinda like black.

C: Like black? The seeds tasted black or they were black?

M: 12. The seeds tasted like black.

C: What do you do on Halloween?

M: 13. Uh my father, he be driving me to people houses. 14. Me and my brother ring the doorbell 15. and we say "Trick or Treat" 16. and it was kids still wearing costumes 17. and the people over Sherri's [listener did not know the identity of this person] house, uh they only got two candies. 18. Yeah, I gonna be Halloween Batman 19. and they did not give me a shirt 20. and I need to go at . . . . um . . . . 21. My mother gonna buy me a shirt at the store. 22. I already got my black pants.

C: Did you see the Batman movie ? [M nods yes] Who was in the movie?

M: 23. Joker.

C: Can you tell me anything about Joker?

M: 24. Uh, well I saw his friends. 25. His friends be white 26. and his friends, pink 27. and they . . . . 28. and his friends be wearing hats and black clothes.

C: What colors did the Joker wear?

M: 29. Um from he like his friend, he, Batman . . . . . put him down in this green stuff.

C: In some green stuff?

M: 30. Like from Joker was like his friends.

C: So he fell into the green stuff. What happened to him after he fell into the green stuff?

M: 31. He turned, he turned into the . . . 32. He got green nails 33. and his hand is white.

C: He looked like he was smiling, huh? Kind of like a clown. What happened at the end of the movie?

M: 34. Uh, Batman, he was looking at a picture 35. and it's like a bat 36. and it's like a light.

C: What happened to the girl in the movie?

M: 37. Well, I know from she's screaming from, from . . . . 38. She saw somebody shoot a man from . . . . 39. She screaming.

C: Did Batman save her?

M: 40. Um, Batman, he just take her, put her in his car and and Batman drive so the Joker can't catch up. 41. Joker in a different car.

Questions

Note: The study of discourse coherence is subjective and will depend upon the listener's familiarity with the speaker and the degree of common knowledge between participants. You will not always agree with my interpretations. Variability in opinion is common with discourse coherence. There is considerable room for different interpretations of utterances.

1. Describe Michael's ability to use the following dimensions of discourse coherence, as described in this section.

Topic maintenance in the following sequences:

Cartoon (utterances 1–8):

Pumpkin pie (9–12):

Halloween (13–22):

Batman movie (23–41):

Informativeness (what information is present and what information is missing?):

Cartoon (1–8):

Halloween (13–22):

Referencing:

Personal referencing (utterances 2, 6, 15, 17, 19):

Fluency (identify these dysfluencies):

Abandoned utterances:

Fillers (Hint: there are three types in this sample. One is the use of um/er. What are the other two fillers that Michael uses? Where are they used?):

Summarize Michael's discourse coherence:

Strengths:

Weaknesses:

Overall discourse coherence (appropriate, inappropriate, or variable, in your opinion):

2. How well will Michael do in school? Support your answer.

3. What intervention goals would you identify for Michael? Why did you select them?

4. It is critical to integrate Michael's intervention with his classroom activities. How would you integrate them?

Part Two

Childhood Language Disorders

Childhood language disorders represent a heterogeneous group of children with a variety of symptoms. There are many perspectives used to study this area (Nelson, 1998; Paul, 2001; Reed, 1994). In this book, two approaches will be highlighted.

The categorical or etiological approach (Bliss, 1985; Nelson, 1998; Paul, 2001) is highlighted in this section. It represents a medical model that includes specific etiological categories of disorders, such as autism, mental retardation, and hearing impairment. It is most often used for educational placements and the provision of other services. This approach is not always useful because it can be difficult to identify a single etiology for a disorder. Disorders may have multiple etiologies. For example, mental retardation and autism frequently co-occur, and the primary cause of the resultant language disorder cannot be specified. The categorical perspective is also limited because unique features are not associated with specific etiologies. There is considerable overlap among disorders and symptoms (Aram & Nation, 1982; Rosenthal, Eisenson, & Luckau, 1972). For example, echolalia is seen not only in autism but in other disorders as well (Schuler, 1979). In addition, children within the same diagnostic category may vary considerably. Etiology is not the sole determinant of language behavior. Social, cultural, economic, emotional, and motivational factors influence language functioning.

A second perspective is based on descriptions of the behaviors or symptoms that a child exhibits; it represents a noncategorical or behavioral approach (Bliss, 1985; Paul, 2001). The focus is not on etiology; behavioral strengths and weaknesses are profiled. A child's developmental level is compared to the sequence of behavior expected in typical language acquisition for a wide range of areas, such as semantics, syntax, morphology, pragmatics, and phonology (Paul, 2001). Significant deviations from typical expectancies would be considered to represent impairments (Paul, 2001). One advantage of this approach is that it enables clinicians to use a broad perspective and not be limited to identifying symptoms that have been considered to be associated with a specific etiology (e.g., echolalia indicates autism). A second advantage is that the information obtained forms the bases of intervention goals (Bliss, 1985). A disadvantage of this approach is that it can be time-consuming; profiling language behavior is a long process. Also, a uniform set of descriptive categories has not been adopted, resulting in different descriptions of behavior, depending upon what clinician evaluated the child (Paul, 2001). In addition, services and educational placements may be difficult to obtain because children are not classified in a way that is readily understood by educators, medical personnel, and professionals in related fields (Paul, 2001). The behavioral approach is used in Parts One and Four of this book.

7
Specific Language Impairment

Children with specific language impairment (SLI) have limited language and communication abilities in comparison to their peers with typical language development of the same chronological age. Approximately 7 percent of preschool children exhibit SLI (Leonard, 1998; Tomblin et al., 1997). Although their nonverbal intelligence is within the average range, they exhibit deficits in symbolic play and auditory processing (Johnston, 1988; Leonard, 1982). Hearing and emotional impairments then are not the cause of their difficulty in learning language. SLI is not a static condition; it changes over time and its effects can be seen even in adulthood (Conti-Ramsden & Botting, 1999; Records, Tomblin, & Freese, 1992).

A major characteristic of SLI is impaired syntactic ability, which may extend through school and adult years (Conti-Ramsden & Botting, 1999; Hadley, 1998a). Use of verb-related forms is particularly vulnerable with respect to copulas, auxiliaries, irregular verbs, and the inflections of third person singular *s* and the past *ed* (Bedore & Leonard, 1998; Bliss, 1985; Conti-Ramsden & Jones, 1997; Goffman & Leonard, 2000; Grela & Leonard, 2000; Leonard, Miller, & Gerber, 1999; Rice, 1994; Rice & Oetting, 1993; Rice & Wexler, 1996). Other syntactic impairments include pronoun substitutions (e.g., *him* for *he*, etc.), rigid use of agents in agent + action + object structures, reduced sentence coordination and embedding, and omission of articles (Bliss, 1985; Lee, 1966).

SLI is not a unitary disorder. It can best be described from the five perspectives described by Leonard (1998). One perspective refers to a simple delay in overall language development. This delay is temporary; by 3 years of age, children have approached typical developmental levels. They are generally not diagnosed as SLI because they have achieved mastery at a relatively early age. They are sometimes described as late talkers (Paul, 2001).

The second perspective is characterized by a plateau in language development. This pattern begins as a delay in the emergence of language forms. It becomes a plateau because development is arrested at an early level; language behaviors are not eventually mastered. A child is "stuck" at an early level of language growth.

A third perspective represents profile differences in the development of language structures. Uneven rates in the development of some features of language structure sometimes occur that cannot be predicted by level of language development. Leonard (1998) provided an example of a profile difference with inflections. Children with typical language development learn the plural *s* before the third-person singular *s*. The difference in the rate of development of these two inflections is expected. Children with SLI show a greater developmental gap between the use of these two inflections than is found in typical development. The third-person singular form is particularly difficult for children with SLI. This pattern suggests a different profile of language development in SLI; there are different degrees of mastery across features of language structure. Another example of a profile difference is evident in the language sample elicited from John that is presented in Chapter 5. His language development is uneven because he has mastered a variety of complex sentences although he has not acquired auxiliaries and articles. This profile appears to be atypical of normal development.

A fourth pattern reflects an abnormal frequency of a specific error. A child with SLI exhibits a specific error that is seen in typical language development but is at a considerably higher rate. An example is the use of the accusative case pronoun for nominative case pronoun. A child might use *me* for *I* or *her* for *she*. While this substitution is seen in typical language development, it is considerably more frequent in SLI.

Finally, a qualitative difference might characterize SLI. This pattern would suggest the use of structures that are not found in typical language development. There are very few examples of this pattern in the research with SLI (Johnston, 1982; Leonard, 1998). An example would be the use of *be* as a pivot in early two-word utterances, as in *be red, be finished* (Lee, 1966).

In the samples for this section, the language patterns of SLI will be compared to those found in typical language development. While it is not always easy to identify a child in one of the patterns described, we will attempt to do so in this section.

Assessment Applications

1. Assessment should consist of comparisons within and across language domains. Clinicians can compare performance among syntax, semantics, morphology, and pragmatics. At more specific levels, comparisons should be made within grammatical categories for noun and verb phrase expansion (e.g., articles versus demonstrative pronouns or auxiliaries versus copulas) and between grammatical categories and grammatical structures (e.g., auxiliaries versus simple and complex sentence use).

2. Verb use is a critical aspect of assessment because this form is vulnerable in SLI (Goffman & Leonard, 2000; Grela & Leonard, 2000).

3. The patterns of impaired language use described by Leonard (1998) should be identified because goals for intervention can be based on these profiles.

Intervention Applications

1. Intervention should generally follow a sequence of typical language development (Fey, 1986).

There are limitations to this developmental approach; it should not be used for every child (see Fey, 1986, for details).

2. Clinicians need to incorporate a variety of structures (e.g., agent + action + object as well as action + object) and a variety of words for each semantic relation (e.g., reference to different agents, actions, and objects) as a means of enhancing flexibility of language use.

3. Group therapy should be implemented whenever possible as a means of fostering social and pragmatic skills, as well as linguistic abilities.

Introduction to Samples

The language samples of two children, matched by MLU, will be compared. MLU was based on a 50-utterance language sample. Both children are in Stage V of language development, when they should begin to use conjoined sentences (Brown, 1973). They would be expected to have mastered auxiliaries and embedded sentences (Brown, 1973). Robert, the child with SLI, has been enrolled in a language intervention program for two years. His language test scores fall two standard deviations below the mean for his chronological age. His nonverbal intelligence level is within average limits. His language usage has not developed spontaneously over several years. His profile has remained consistent.

Lindsay and Robert

Lindsay

2 years, 10 months, MLU 4.06 (based on 50-utterance sample)

Adult: Let's make something in the sand.

Lindsay: 1. What that? (points to tape recorder)

A: That's a tape recorder.

L: 2. Cathy you got any little baby?

A: All I have is a husband.

L: 3. I have husband. 4. I got my mommy . . . . . 5. Have that at your house? . . . .

A: No not yet.

L: 6. I know but that your sandcastle. 7. This is my sandcastle . . . 8. Have doggie at your house?

A: No. We can't. I'm allergic to dogs.

L: 9. You have allergic . . . 10. Want one (some sand) Cathy? 11. I dump all out.

A: What's your dog's name?

L: 12. Brandy, he's a doggie. 13. I got pockets (shows adult the pockets on her dress).

A: Just like mine.

L: 14. You go in my wagon?

A: I'm too big.

L: 15. You can go on my bike.

A: I'm too big for your bike too.

L: [rides her bike] 16. This is pedal. 17. This is wheel. 18. Turn and you ride it.

A: You're riding in a circle.

L: 19. I got two rubber band for on my bike. 20. Are you watching? 21. I gonna get Brandy.

A: Let's play here.

L: 22. What this?

A: A tape recorder

L: 23. What these?

A: A shoe.

L: 24. I know what them. 25. That's my doggie.

A: She's a nice dog.

L: 26. Her name Brandy. 27. Let's go down [to] play in water. 28. My hair's long too. 29. This is bucket [of] water. 30. You got baby?

A: No

L: 31. Do you have crib?

A: No, I have a bed.

L: 32. I got my own bed.

Robert

6 years, 0 months, MLU 4.26 (based on 50-utterance sample)

Adult: Aren't you tired? [from running up the stairs]

Robert: 33. Me tired. 34. What's that? 35. We gonna talk in that? [tape recorder]

A: Yes. Later we'll play it back so you can hear yourself. We're going to play a game.

R: 36. Why kids go in this room?

A: Don't you have a speech room you go to?

R: 37. Yeah, it painted.

A: How do you like summer camp?

R: 38. Me like some of it.

A: What do you like to do the best?

R: 39. Go swimming.

A: Are you a good swimmer?

R: 40. Me don't swim under water. 41. Me drown under there.

A: Can you hold your breath for a long time?

R: 42. Me don't swim very well. 43. Me know how to swim. 44. Why this rocks? [points to chair he is sitting on]

A: It might be broken.

R: 45. Broke?

A: It might have broken springs.

R: 46. Me can't see spring.

A: I can't seem them either. What sticker do you want?

R: 47. Me want this one.

A: Do you like stickers?

R: [trying to peel it off backing paper] 48. Will this come off?

A: Sure, do you want to put it on your shirt?

R: 49. Can't pull it off.

A: What do you do right here in this room?

R: 50. Games and papers. 51. Me got notebook.

A: You got your own notebook!

R: 52. Me made it.

A: Here's a picture of a bird. Do you have a bird at home?

R: 53. Mine dead.

A: Did someone run over it?

R: 54. No, snake bite it.

A: Oh dear, that's too bad. Did you go to the parade yesterday?

R: 55. Me went. 56. You didn't go?

A: No. How do you like living will all of the kids?

R: 57. Me don't like to eat there.

A: What does your speech teacher do with you?

R: 58. Get mean to me.

A: Why does he get mean?

R: 59. 'Cause me don't be good.

A: You're not good? Let's play with these fishing poles and fish.

R: 60. What you gonna have, close pins? [are safety pins]

A: You want to go fishing?

R: 61. That a real fishing pole? 62. How you do that?

A: Yeah, do you want to see my fish?

R: 63. Yeah, what you do? 64. That them real fishies.

Questions

1. Review the five patterns of SLI and determine which pattern is best able to describe Robert.

2. **a.** Compare Robert and Lindsay with respect to the use of the personal pronoun *I*, copulas, articles, and complex sentences. Which child is more advanced? Why?

Pronoun *I*:

Copulas:

Articles:

Complex sentences:

   b. Is Robert functioning at the same language level as Lindsay, even though they have similar MLUs? Support your answer.

3. What are the intervention goals for Robert?

4. What are the therapy implications of each pattern of SLI?

   a. Delay in development:

   b. Plateau in development:

   c. Profile differences among aspects of language structure:

   d. Abnormally high frequency of an error:

   e. Qualitative difference in usage:

5. Many doctors tell parents of children who are late talkers not to worry about their child's slowness. They do not recommend that the parents consult with a speech-language pathologist. They say that the child will outgrow the delay in talking. What could you say to a doctor to change this standard advice?

8

Language Learning Disorders in Adolescence

The language disorders of preschool and elementary school frequently become more subtle in adolescence (Nippold, 1988). Approximately 50 percent of adolescents with a history of specific language impairment have academic difficulties and require special education (Strothard, Snowling, Bishop, Chipchase, & Kaplan, 1998). They cannot meet the academic challenges of the classroom (Ehrens, 1994; Whitmire, 2000). The disorders are often difficult to identify because the symptoms vary and are discreet (Nelson, 1988). The term *language learning disorder* is used to reflect the language basis of the impairment that occurs in adolescence.

Language learning impairments in adolescents are characterized by a variety of deficits. Adolescents may be reduced in their abstract thought processes and problem-solving skills (Wiig, 1995). There may be an overreliance on literal meanings, resulting in limited ability to understand ambiguity, metaphors, similes, puns and proverbs (Nippold, 1988). Advanced phonological processing abilities, such as repeating complex words and phrases, may be limited (Kamhi & Catts, 1989). Also, reading and writing impairments may be evident (Kamhi & Catts, 1989; Nelson, 1998). Discourse coherence deficits are evident. Social impairments result in the inability to relate to peers and other individuals (Ehrens, 1994; Whitmire, 2000).

Many adolescents have word-finding difficulties that accompany a learning disability (German, 1987; German & Simon, 1991; Wiig & Semel, 1984). This deficit is evident in spontaneous naming tasks (also called confrontation naming) and is frequently associated with dysflluent production in discourse (German, 1987; German & Simon, 1991). The dysfluencies described in Chapter 6 (e.g., abandoned utterances, internal corrections, repetitions, pauses, and fillers) are frequently evident in the discourse of children with language learning disabilities. Children with word-retrieval deficits also use circumlocutions to describe an intended word. Semantic or phonological lexical substitutions may also be evident (McGregor, 1997). Word-retrieval deficits may result from an inability to access a word or a limited knowledge of a word (Kail & Leonard, 1986; Leonard, Nippold, Kail, & Hale, 1983).

A language disorder in adolescence has a negative impact on major aspects of life, including personal, social, vocational, and economic adjustment (Reed, 1994). Adolescents with language learning disorders encounter many social problems (Whitmire, 2000). They have difficulty resisting peer pressure, do not participate in class discussions, and are generally not motivated to improve their academic and communicative skills (Ehrens, 1994).

Assessment of adolescent language disorders needs to be multifaceted. Traditional syntactic analyses are not generally informative because adolescents have acquired most syntactic forms (Scott, 1988; Scott & Stokes, 1995). Focus on late-developing syntactic structures is unproductive because these structures occur infrequently in discourse (Scott & Stokes, 1995). Discourse analyses are more revealing. However, conversation is too simple for most adolescents with a language learning disorder; deficits may not be revealed in this genre. Narrative discourse is useful for assessment because it enables clinicians to focus on event sequencing as well as topic maintenance and referencing. Expository discourse is also important to evaluate. It consists of descriptions and explanations of phenomena, reports, argumentation, and persuasion (Larson & McKinley, 1995; Nelson, 1998; Paul, 2001). Its purpose is to transmit information. Expository discourse is used frequently in the classroom; it is a more demanding discourse genre than narration (Scott & Windsor, 2000).

In this section, conversational discourse is analyzed because the sample reveals significant difficulties that the speaker has with this genre. Narrative and expository discourse samples could also have been elicited and analyzed from this adolescent speaker.

Assessment Applications

1. Assessment of the language behavior of adolescents should be expanded to include dimensions that would not be measured with younger children, such as knowledge of language structure (e.g., metalinguistics), thought processes (e.g., metacognition), and discourse (e.g., metapragmatics). Verbal reasoning, problem-solving abilities, reading, and writing should also be assessed (Kamhi & Catts, 1989; Paul, 2001; Nelson, 1998; Nippold, 1988, 2000; Scott, 1988; Scott & Stokes, 1995; Wiig, 1995).

2. Social skills and word-retrieval abilities also need to be assessed.

3. The motivations of the adolescent to improve communicative abilities should be considered. Clinicians need to identify what will motivate an adolescent to improve communicative performance (e.g., effective discourse coherence for job interviews or social situations).

Intervention Applications

1. Motivation is difficult to achieve with adolescents; they frequently do not want to be singled out for treatment and often do not understand the negative impact of their communicative disorder (Larson & McKinley, 1995). To overcome reduced motivation, the clinician should incorporate materials and contexts that are related to the lives and interests of an adolescent, such as employment, social skills, and money (Larson & McKinley, 1995).

2. Generalization of skills needs to be directly incorporated in an intervention program. Use of natural contexts (e.g., gymnasium and cafeteria settings) and a variety of discourse genres (e.g., narratives) will be expected to facilitate generalization to social situations (Nippold, 2000). Transitions need to be made from the intervention program to the classroom.

3. Increasing phonological processing abilities as well as metacognitive and metalinguistic knowledge are integral components of a program for adolescents (Larson & McKinley, 1995).

Introduction to the Sample

Rudy has been enrolled in a language intervention program in a public school. He scored within the average range on a standardized intelligence test. His language test scores were two standard deviations below the mean for his chronological age.

Rudy

14 years

Clinician: What are you looking for?

Rudy: 1. Just lost a black marker.

C: Did you leave it here or did you take it home last night?

R: 2. Leave it here [points to his desk], my desk like by these other books. 3. Well, it was kinda like by the middle. 4. These one book, like over here [points], and then these other books over here [points to a different location] 5. and like the janitor always move my desk around 6. and I put over there [pointing to a location in the front of the classroom] 7. and I thinking the . . . . . maybe janitor moving it. 8. The marker must have fell.

C: The janitor moves your desk around at night?

R: 9. Well, mostly my desk 10. because most of the time I move my desk 11. because it has to be like by uh kinda by uh in front of these books. 12.

Then um a kid came I don't like 13. so I move down. 14. So then it was this table in back of me 15. and I keep on moving it like all the time 16. and I get up . . . . 17. I like sometimes accidentally move my chair like that [moves his chair to demonstrate] and get up 18. but mostly I have to go like this [pushes desk away]. 19. When my desk . . . . .20. and then get up.

C: So you think when you moved your desk, maybe the pen fell out?

R: 21.Well you move the desk yeah. 22. Well before that, stuff happens. 23. Like in school there is like move my desk all the way back. 24. I could . . . .25. and then my teacher made me move my desk by these book 26. and yesterday um . . .27. The books are like a lot. 28. They they move it 29. and then you like in front of my way 30. I couldn't see my teacher 31. so I moved down 32. and then I decided to move down more. 33. I could see the umm umm the map.

C: You wanted to be able to see your teacher?

R: 34. Yeah and the map 35. and that because the map was over here 36. and I was over there [points to a location in the room].

Questions

1. Rudy's deficits are primarily in the area of discourse rather than syntax. Describe his performance (Appropriate? Inappropriate? Variable?) with respect to the following dimensions of discourse and justify your answers:

Topic Maintenance:

Informativeness:

Referencing:

Appropriate use:

Inappropriate use:

Fluency:

2. What intervention goals would be appropriate for Rudy?

3. What communication behaviors will be difficult for Rudy in his classroom (e.g., following complex directions)?

4. Social impairments are also evident in adolescent language learning disorders. What impairments in social interaction might an adolescent with language learning disorders exhibit?

9

Mental Retardation

Mental retardation is characterized by a deficit in age-appropriate adaptive behavior and below-average cognitive functioning. There is considerable individual variation among individuals with mental retardation, resulting from differences in etiology (e.g., genetic disorders versus brain injury), intellectual functioning, and social experiences. The levels of retardation, with respect to intellectual quotient (IQ), are: mild or educable (IQ between 52–68), moderate or trainable (IQ between 36–51), severe (IQ between 20–35), and profound (IQ below 20) (Grossman, 1983). Children with mild (e.g., educable) retardation function independently in society while children with moderate retardation need some adult supervision but are able to communicate adequately. Individuals at the lower two levels have speech, language, and communicative impairments and need supervision (Grossman, 1983).

Significant language impairments are not evident in children whose IQs are above 55 (Owens, 1997). Some language and discourse impairments that are evident in children with IQs below 55 are short simple sentences, limited use of adjectives and adverbs, errors in subject-verb agreement and other grammatical categories, concrete vocabulary, limited requests for clarification, and reduced assertiveness (Lackner, 1968; Owens, 1997).

The relationship between cognition and language is not completely understood, however, they influence each other (Cromer, 1991; Piaget, 1926; Vygotsky, 1962.) Factors other than IQ—such as motivation, personality, and experience—influence language and communicative behavior (Kamhi & Johnston, 1982; Leahy, Balla, & Zigler, 1982). Poor performance on intelligence tests may reflect limited attention span or distractibility (Leahy, Balla, & Zigler, 1982). Test scores do not reflect the social capabilities of individuals. Clinicians need to consider many factors that influence communicative functioning.

Assessment Applications

1. A test score that yields mental age or IQ should not be the only predictor of communicative functioning. Personality and social experience need to be considered.

2. Language test scores need to be supplemented with language samples and observations of behavior. Children's test scores may not be indicative of their functional communication.

3. Communicative functioning should be assessed in different contexts (e.g., home, classroom, recess, and lunch) and with different partners (e.g., peers, siblings, and teachers).

Intervention Applications

1. Communicative functioning should be the first priority when working with individuals with mental retardation. Syntax should receive secondary focus when communication is impaired.

2. Generalization needs to be a primary goal in intervention (Owens, 1997). Generalization is fostered by working outside an intervention setting and using different contexts and conversational partners.

3. Some individuals with mental retardation are passive conversationalists; they use more responsive than assertive conversational acts. For these individuals, increased use of assertive conversational acts such as requests for information or action, commands and directions, as well as comments should be targeted (see Chapter 2 for details on these conversational acts).

Introduction to Samples

Eddy is enrolled in a classroom for children with educable mental retardation. His nonverbal intelligence quotient is 65. He is 11 years and 5 months old. Ted is enrolled in a classroom for children with trainable mental retardation. His nonverbal intelligence quotient is 48. He is 11 years old.

The two samples are unequal in length. Eddy's sample showed more variability; more utterances were needed to reveal the range of his utterances. Ted's sample was more consistent; fewer utterances were needed to reveal the trends evident in language use.

Eddy and Ted

Eddy

Enrolled in a classroom for children with educable mental retardation

11 years, 5 months

Eddy: 1. Um, I know how to work the VCR.

Clinician: You've known how to work that for a long time.

E: 2. Yep, I got the new movie couple weeks ago.

C: What movie?

E: 3. *Land Before Time.*

C: What happens?

E: 4. Um, them, um them looking for the great valley. 5. I don't know what um Petrie did 6. and and I think I don't know what the other one did. 7. I played, um I went to Blockbusters. 8. My mom bought me a movie, a film.

C: What movie?

E: 9. I watched *Freddy's Nightmares.*

C: Was it scary?

E: 10. No, it about a lady who kill her husband 11. then . . . . her found letters . . . . 12. In the ending her fall down. 13. Somebody sat down, 14. fall down 15. fall down off a ladder. 16. I watched *Friday the 13th Part 6* this summer.

C: You watch a lot of scary movies. You're not scared of them?

E: 17. No . . . I play outside this summer. 18. I went in the swimming pool. 19. I, I saw a . . . 20. I went to the fire station house, open house.

C: You did? Did they show you how fast firemen have to get dressed for fires?

E: 21. No, but them show us um climb the ladder.

C: What else did they show you?

E: 22. One fireman tell me something.

C: What did he tell you?

E: 23. First you gotta be good in school and go high school. 24. Then go to the other high school and work good. 25. Then teach a fireman . . . . 26. Then them pick um a good firemans.

C: Remember when you came and saw me up at school? That was kinda far away. I don't go there anymore.

E: 27. Why? 28. You got fired?

C: No, I graduated.

E: 29. When?

C: This past June.

E: 30. When you get your driving lesson?

C: I've had my driver's license since I was in high school.

E: 31. You flunk?

C: No.

E: 32. Only once?

C: I never flunked my driver license test.

E: 33. Never? 34. Um Never you flunk?

C: I never flunked.

E: 35. What you didn't? 36. What do you did?

C: I don't think I ever flunked. I might have flunked a test.

E: 37. You flunked your driving test?

C: No.

E: 38. What you did?

C: What did I do, you mean for my driver's license?

E: 39. Yes.

Ted

Enrolled in a classroom for children with trainable mental retardation

11 years, 3 months

Clinician: What are you gonna do on the picnic?

T: 40. Well, uh I . . . I do run.

C: Are you gonna do anything else?

T: 41. Well, I do eat sandwich.

C: How are you gonna get to the picnic?

T: 42. My mom's got a car at home.

C: You're gonna go with her?

T: 43. No, I going to picnic Tuesday.

C: You went to the Special Olympics? What did you do there?

T: 44. Well, we was . . . I was runnin' fast.

C: What else happened there?

T: 45. Well, we do . . . uh . . . I fixed . . . 46. We do play baseball.

C: Did you win?

T: 47. No, I . . . I was got two . . . two shots.

C: Are you gonna go to the Special Olympics next year?

T: 48. Yeah, no, I . . . I going to the camp.

C: What activities are there at camp?

T: 49. Well . . . we do um there . . . we do . . . I do play some um . . . 50. I fix . . . .

C: Did you just come from your class? [Ted nods] What were you working on in class?

T: 51. We do color and we do our names.

C: Do you play?

T: 52. I do play at home.

C: What's your favorite thing to play with?

T: 53. Uh . . . well . . . I fixed pick-up the cars. 54. Um I fix trucks.

C: How do you fix a truck?

T: 55. Well, I do put some parts on it. 56. I go home.

C: Do you help your mom cook at home?

T: 57. Yeah, sometimes I do.

C: How do you do that?

T: 58. My mom do put some . . . some dinner in there. 59. I do make . . . help him . . . her.

C: I bet you are a good helper.

T: 60. Yeah, My mom . . . my mom got a pot.

C: What does she do with the pot?

T: 61. Put something in . . . in the pot.

C: What does she put in the pot?

T: 62. Salt.

C: What do you do with salt?

T: 63. I do shake it.

C: What are you gonna do this weekend?

T: 64. Well, I doin' next . . . this, this weekend . . . 65. I gonna go . . . 66. I gotta plant plants.

C: You gotta plant plants?

T: 67. Yea, plant for my friend next week.

C: Why are you gonna do that?

T: 68. They are my friends.

Questions

1. Which child is a more active conversationalist? Look at asking questions and initiating new topics. Support your answer.

2. Eddy and Ted have difficulty with some syntactic forms. Compare each child with respect to:

   a. The presence and absence of the auxiliary *do* in each child's sample
      Eddy:

      Ted:

   b. Use of the pronouns *she* and *they*
      Eddy:

      Ted:

   c. Use of complex sentences
      Eddy:

      Ted:

3. Overall, which child's language development is more advanced? Why?

4. What would be your intervention goals for Eddy and Ted? Consider syntax and/or discourse. Justify your answer.

5. Children with mental retardation frequently have difficulty generalizing what they have learned in a structured clinical context to a more unstructured functional setting (Owens, 1997). What procedures could be implemented in intervention to foster generalization?

10
Autism

Autism (or autistic spectrum disorder) is an impairment within the larger category of pervasive developmental disorders (American Psychiatric Association, 1994). It is primarily characterized by impaired social interaction and communicative functioning. There is heterogeneity within the group of individuals who are diagnosed with autism. Mental retardation accompanies autism for some individuals; others have average or even above-average intelligence. Some individuals, especially those with average intelligence, have appropriate syntactic abilities (Long, 1994).

Echolalia is a primary symptom of autism (Long, 1994; Tiegerman-Farber, 1997). It consists of the repetition of words and phrases that have been spoken by another individual (Prizant & Duchan, 1981). It is found in approximately 75 percent of children with autism and is also evident in other disorders, such as severe language impairment, mental retardation, blindness, brain injury, and neurological deficits (Schuler, 1979).

There are two types of echolalia. Immediate echolalia is characterized by a relatively brief latency between a previous utterance and a repeated one (Long, 1994). An example is:

Adult: *Pick up the red one*. Child: *Red one*.

Frequently the last word or words of an utterance are repeated, as a means of understanding or processing the previous utterance.

The second type is delayed echolalia. The latency is greater than with immediate echolalia and may even span days or weeks (Long, 1994). For example, a child with autism was facing three elevator doors. He pointed to one elevator and said, *Behind door number one*—a phrase he had heard on a television show. The child could produce only a few one-word utterances; the echo was more advanced than his spontaneous language behavior. The meaning and intent of a delayed echo will partially depend upon the listener's

familiarity with a child and with the context (Prizant & Rydell, 1984). Individuals familiar with the child may have a better understanding of the delayed echo.

Both immediate and delayed echolalia consist of exact repetitions or modifications (e.g., mitigated echolalia) of an original utterance. Children who have modifications in their echoic responses have higher intelligence levels, more advanced language development, and a better prognosis for further development than children whose utterances do not have modifications (Fay & Butler, 1968). With mitigated echolalia, children appear to be processing the previous utterance. Children may be echoing as a means of trying to understand the utterance.

Echolalia is selective. Children with severe impairments do not repeat all the utterances that they hear (Fay, 1967; Fay & Schuler, 1980). Linguistic and pragmatic factors influence echolalia. Children repeat more open-ended questions than questions that require one-word answers (Fay, 1975). Statements elicit more echoes than commands or questions (Matheny, 1968). Words that are not known to a child tend to be echoed (Violette & Swisher, 1992). Comprehension deficits are frequently related to echolalia. Utterances that exceed the comprehension level of a speaker are often repeated (Carr, Schreibman, & Lovaas, 1975; Fay & Schuler, 1980; Rutter, 1968). However, some utterances that a child understands are repeated (Paccia, Cooper, & Curcio, 1979). We do not understand completely why some utterances are repeated and others are not (Fay & Schuler, 1980).

Traditionally, echolalia has been considered an aberrant and meaningless behavior (Fay & Schuler, 1980; Rutter, 1968). More recently, investigators have determined that immediate and delayed echolalic utterances serve communicative and/or cognitive functions (Prizant & Duchan, 1981; Prizant & Rydell, 1984). The communicative functions of turn taking, requesting, gaining attention, and stating and answering characterize immediate and delayed echolalia (Prizant & Duchan, 1981; Prizant & Rydell,

1984). Cognitive functions of echolalia include rehearsal, self-regulation, and self-direction (Prizant & Duchan, 1981; Prizant & Rydell, 1984). Both immediate and delayed echolalia should be viewed on a continuum of functions, consisting of comprehension ability, exactness of repetition, and perceived communicative intent (Prizant & Rydell, 1984).

Assessment Applications

1. Patterns of echolalia should be identified by answering the following questions: Does a child echo more statements than questions? Are there more echoes with complex stimuli than simple sentences? and Does a child echo utterances that have abstract, rather than concrete, vocabulary?

2. The functions of echolalia should be identified, as in communicative (e.g., turn taking, requesting, gaining attention, stating and answering) and cognitive (e.g., rehearsal, self-regulation, and self-direction) uses.

3. Clinicians need to assess the comprehension abilities of a child who echoes frequently.

Intervention Applications

1. If a pattern of echolalia can be identified, an intervention hierarchy can be established. The clinician begins where the child does not echo and gradually increases complexity toward the types of utterances that the child tends to repeat.

2. Comprehension abilities should be improved if there are impairments in this modality.

3. Parents and teachers need to be advised regarding the nature of echolalia—that it is not a willful act of noncompliance. They should be counseled to respond to the communicative intent of a child's echoed utterance.

Introduction to the Samples

In this section, immediate and delayed echolalia will be compared. Evan is severely language impaired. He is enrolled in a language remediation preschool program for children with autism. Kevin is enrolled in a special education class for children with autism.

Immediate Echolalia

Evan
4 years, 6 months

The clinician and child are playing in a therapy room with play dough. There are other toys in a paper bag near them.

Clinician: I just made a ball [playing with play dough].

Evan: 1. Made a ball?

C: Yeah, can you make something?

E: 2. I make a ball.

C: Ok.

E: 3. Make it like . . . making it.

C: This is kind of stiff play dough because it's brand new. There's a ball for you. It looks kind of like a snowball.

E: 4. Snowball.

C: What else is in the bag?

E: 5. A can.

C: It's another color.

E: 6. Another color.

C: Do you know what color that is?

E: 7. Yeah, that can.

C: It's blue.

E: 8. It's blue.

C: I'll make a snake.

E: 9. I make a snake.

C: My snake broke in two.

E: 10. Is top [putting one piece of play dough on top of another].

C: I made a bracelet.

E: 11. Bracelet.

C: Oh no! Look, my bracelet is breaking.

E: 12. Is bracelet?

C: I'll take it off now.

E: 13. What in there?

C: More of this stuff [play dough].

E: 14. More stuff [takes out another can of play dough].

C: Would you like to make a house?

E: 15. Make a house.

C: What color is this house?

E: 16. This color house.

C: It's red.

E: 17. Red.

C: We'll make it a red house. What color is the roof?

E: 18. Color roof.

C: Is it white? [the roof is red]

E: 19. White.

C: I'll make a square house.

E: 20. Square house.

C: It looks like a snowman. It doesn't look like a house. Here's his head.

E: 21. Gotta make bounce ball [forms the play dough into a ball].

C: A bouncing ball. Will it bounce?

E: 22. Yeah.

C: I don't know if play dough bounces or not.

E: 23. This ball bounce.

C: What color do you have? I'll get the white. I'll put away the blue.

E: 24. Put the top in it.

C: Yeah, we have to put the top on it or it will dry out.

E: 25. Dry out.

C: We still have more. What can does that go in?

E: 26. That go in.

C: I have some more toys in here. [bag with toys] Wanna see what's in there?

E: 27. Yeah, what this?

C: What is it, you know?

E: 28. Bunny.

C: That's right. Like at Easter time.

E: 29. What that? [looks at a bag of toys.]

C: It's a bird.

E: 30. A bird.

C: What are you going to make?

E: 31. People [gets out small cooking pan].

C: Are you going to cook some lunch?

E: 32. Cook some lunch.

C: What are we going to have?

E: 33. Dinner.

C: Dinner?

E: 34. Some cook [puts play dough in a pan and stirs].

C: It looks like white soup.

E: 35. White soup.

Delayed Echolalia

Kevin
11 years, 3 months

Kevin has been talking about Super Mario Brothers Three, a video game.

Kevin: 1. Now it's Beetlejuice . . . . ghost with the most.

Clinician: Who's Beetlejuice?

K: 2. He's the one ghost with the most.

C: What does he do?

K: 3. America, America's number-one ghost with the most.

C: Who is that?

K: 4. He's Nintendo Entertainment System.

C: What does Beetlejuice do, Kevin?

K: 5. He jumps under the sea.

C: Oh.

K: 6. And he sees the mermaid and then Beetlejuice gonna rescue Lidia.

C: Who's Lidia?

K: 7. The one for the one Beetlejuice. 8. It's a . . . it's a . . . . and the Saturday morning. 9. Now he's Nintendo Entertainment System.

C: Where?

K: 10. Nintendo Entertainment System.

C: What's your favorite game on Nintendo?

K: 11. He gonna find Super Mario Brothers Three.

C: That's your favorite one. Why do you like Super Mario Brothers Three the best?

K: 12. This one, the number [points to the chalkboard, where he has written, "Super Mario Brothers Three"]. 13. And two [writes on the chalkboard and the clinician reaches for the chalk]. 14. I not finished yet.

C: Can you tell me abut Super Mario Brothers Three?

K: 15. Beetlejuice gonna find one 16. and then Beetlejuice gonna find a real two.

C: What does Beetlejuice do?

K: 17. He swims.

C: How abut other video games? What other ones do you have?

K: 18. He gonna find another Super Mario Brothers Two.

C: Who?

K: 19. Beetlejuice. 20. If Beetlejuice find Nintendo Entertainment System . . . . 21. Beetlejuice of the Lost Nintendo. 22. That's why Beetlejuice goon find . . . he gonna find the World of Nintendo.

C: What does he have to find?

K: 23. The World of Nintendo 24. And that's the ghost with the most and he says, "Hey, hey I XXXX you to death." 25. When he, when he's behind, she behind him. 26. Beetlejuice keep walk and walk . . . . 27. He gonna find . . .

C: He gonna find Nintendo?

K: 28. Uhuh [yes]. 29. Book belong to Miss N [his teacher].

C: What book?

K: 30. Belong to Miss N.

C: Which one?

K: 31. This book [points to clinician's pad of paper].

Questions (for Evan's sample)

1. Identify the 18 echolalic utterances in Evan's sample.

2. Provide support for the claim that Evan has limitations in understanding the word, *color,* and the concepts it represents.

3. Does Evan echo more statements than questions? What is the significance of this finding regarding Evan's communicative competence?

4. What intervention goals would you have for Evan?

Questions (for Kevin's sample)

1. Identify the different examples (e.g., themes or topics) of delayed echolalia (chunks of memorized forms).

2. What would be your intervention goals for Kevin?

3. Do you think Evan or Kevin is more communicatively impaired? Why?

4. In your opinion, does the language development evident in autism reflect a delay or a qualitatively different pattern of development? Why?

5. It is critical for the professional to provide information regarding echolalia to the significant others of a child with autism. What information do you need to provide about echolalia to parents and teachers?

11

Hearing Impairment

Children with hearing impairment (HI) exhibit a broad range of language and communication deficits (Quigley, 1978; Quigley & Paul, 1984; Radziewicz & Antonellis, 1997; Shaw, 1994). Factors that are related to the language development of individuals with HI are degree of hearing loss, age of onset and identification of hearing loss, type of loss, and age and type of amplification and education (Quigley & Kretschmer, 1982). The following hearing threshold levels have been used to classify hearing acuity in the best ear: 0–15 dB, normal; 16–25 dB, slight hearing loss; 26–40 dB, mild hearing loss; 41–65 dB, moderate hearing loss; 65–95 dB, severe hearing loss; 96+ dB, profound hearing loss (Northern & Downs, 1984).

Losses above 40 dB will result in noticeable speech and language impairments (Northern & Downs, 1991). Mild losses have a negative impact on academic achievement and social interaction (Shaw, 1994). Acuity will be a major factor in language development with higher levels of hearing loss.

Studies of the syntactic abilities of school-aged and college students have frequently involved analyses of writing because of the limited speech intelligibility of many individuals with severe and profound losses (Quigley, Power, & Stenkamp, 1977; Quigley, Smith, & Wilbur, 1974; Russell, Quigley & Power, 1976). However, writing abilities do not necessarily reflect oral proficiency. Some individuals with severe and profound hearing impairments have written atypical syntactic structures on a test of language knowledge (Quigley, Smith, & Wilbur, 1974). These forms reflect impairments in writing and may not be apparent in oral language behavior. Unfortunately, limited speech intelligibility prevents a thorough understanding of the oral abilities of individuals with severe and profound hearing losses.

The syntactic language behavior of children with HI with moderate and above losses is generally characterized by overuse of simple sentences; limited conjoined and embedded sentences; rigid speaking style; and reduced function words, adjectives, adverbs, and inflections (Quigley & Paul, 1984; Radziewicz & Antonellis, 1997; Russell, Quigley, & Power, 1976). Their utterances have the appearance of telegraphic speech, with a predominance of nouns and verbs, especially at the more severe levels of hearing impairment. Language development is characterized as delayed, with emergence of structures in the same order as found in typical language development (Quigley, Power, & Stenkamp, 1977; Shaw, 1994).

Deficits are observed in semantic ability. Children with moderate to severe hearing impairments tend to have reduced vocabulary (Radziewicz & Antonellis, 1997). They have difficulty understanding abstract concepts and figurative meanings. Concepts such as size and space, which are perceived by sight, are acquired more easily than other concepts, such as time (Shaw, 1994). Severity of loss tends to influence vocabulary and concept attainment (Shaw, 1994).

Impairments in discourse have been observed from preschool through the school years. Reduced initiating and maintaining conversations are evident in both oral and manual communication modes (McKirdy & Blank 1982; Weiss, 1986). Deficits in turn taking, repair strategies, clarification requests, and topic management have been reported (Shaw, 1994). Children with hearing impairments will most likely encounter difficulties in engaging in conversations in mainstreamed classrooms (Weiss, 1986). Their narratives are unelaborated and reduced in concept development (Yoshinaga-Itano, 1986). In adolescence, when communication and peer relationships are critical, difficulties may be encountered (Stinson & Whitmire, 2000). Adolescents with hearing impairments and limited oral communication tend to feel more of a sense of isolation in regular classrooms than in separate schools because they are limited in communicating with their hearing peers (Stinson & Whitmire, 2000).

Children with hearing impairments exhibit academic deficiencies as well. In particular, reading, writing, and spelling are impaired (Nelson, 1998). To compound their academic difficulties, they do not make clarification requests to obtain information that they have missed. In my experience, it has been difficult to encourage students with HI to request information. They appear to want to mask their comprehension deficits.

American Sign Language (ASL) may also be used to assess the abilities of children with hearing impairments. ASL is a rule-governed language system that is used by many individuals with severe and profound hearing impairments.

Assessment Applications

1. A major obstacle in assessment with individuals with moderate and above hearing loss is their reduced speech intelligibility. Clinicians should seek the assistance of an individual who is familiar with the person to help them understand the speaker.

2. Deaf clients may need to be assessed in American Sign Language (ASL) to determine their true capabilities.

3. Reading and writing abilities should not be assumed to reflect oral production and comprehension abilities.

Intervention Applications

1. Speech intelligibility needs primary focus if an oral approach is used, involving speech sound production, intonation, and resonance. American Sign Language may be a viable alternative for some individuals with severe and profound hearing impairments.

2. Concept development (e.g., size, color, causality, and temporal and spatial relations) should be fostered if this is an area of weakness.

3. Flexibility of production needs to be stressed because many children with moderate to severe HI produce rigid structures. Children should be encouraged to use different sentence structures (e.g., questions, negatives, and complex sentences) to vary their sentence structure.

Introduction to Sample

Mark is 9 years old. He has a severe sensorineural hearing loss. The acuity in his better ear ranges from 80 to 90 dB. He wears bilateral hearing aids. He is in an oral training program, learning to speak and read lips. His speech is difficult to understand unless the listener knows what he is talking about. A clinician familiar with Mark elicited and transcribed this sample.

Hearing Impairment
Mark
9 years, 10 months

Clinician: How was school today?

Mark: 1. We ate hot dogs at school and I went to gym.

C: Did you have gym outside today?

M: 2. No, in school.

C: What did you play in gym?

M: 3. We played baseball. 4. Robbie was pitcher. 5. I was catcher. 6. I hit home run [gestures to show a ball going high].

C: Did your teacher play in gym with you?

M: 7. No, too fat.

C: Where is your mother?

M: 8. Mother is in the car.

C: Do you drive a car?

M: 9. No, too small.

C: Would you like to drive a car?

M: 10. Yes, I drive fast [gestures a car crash].

C: How did you hurt your knee?

M: 11. I was riding my bike.

C: How did you fall down?

M: 12. Sheldon push me off my bike.

C: Then what happened?

M: 13. Fell down.

C: Who won your last baseball game?

M: 14. My team won the game.

C: Did you get to play?

M: 15. Uhuh [nods yes], hit the ball two times.

C: When are you going camping?

M: 16. I don't know, in June, July.

C: Where is your father?

M: 17. Father is at the store. 18. He came home at 7 o'clock. 19. Tomorrow Sheldon and Mark go to the store.

C: Do you work at the store on Saturdays?

M: 20. Sheldon work at the store. 21. I go sometimes. 22. I carry boxes.

Questions

1. Evaluate Mark's syntactic development for noun and verb phrase elaboration and complex sentence usage (note that he uses a variety of inflectional word endings).

Articles

   present:

   absent:

Copulas

   present:

   absent:

Auxiliaries

   present:

   absent:

Presence of modals:

Presence of adjectives before a noun:

Presence of complex sentences:

2. Mark's sentence production is rigid. Support this claim.

3. Mark also uses ellipsis, a speaking style in which redundant information is deleted (Halliday & Hassan, 1976). Ellipsis is expected in typical conversations in order to avoid redundancy; it usually occurs in response to questions. However, with Mark, there is an overuse of ellipsis. He shortens his responses and focuses only on a salient aspect of production. Where are his elliptical utterances? What is the effect of Mark's ellipsis on his production?

4. What would be your goals in intervention for Mark?

5. Would Mark benefit from a manual approach to communication in your opinion? Support your answer.

12
Traumatic Brain Injury

Traumatic brain injury (TBI) is common in young adults between the ages of 15 and 24 years, resulting from car and sports accidents, falls, and, for infants, physical abuse (Beukelman & Yorkston, 1991). The external injury to the brain results in cognitive, communicative, behavioral, emotional, and motor impairments (Ylvisaker & Szekeres, 1989). Individuals with TBI represent a diverse population. Their level of functioning is dependent upon many factors, including severity and locus of damage, length of time in a coma, amount of posttraumatic amnesia, age, medical status, and behavioral and personality variables (Ewing-Cobbs, Fletcher, & Levin, 1985).

Syntactic abilities are generally preserved in TBI because the speech and language centers in the brain are not damaged (Ylvisaker & Feeney, 1995). Utterance length, sentence complexity, and grammaticality are typically appropriate (Turkstra & Holland, 1998).

Executive functions, which are associated with prefontal lobe activity in the brain, are often impaired. Executive functions include establishing goals; initiating, planning, or organizing relevant behaviors to meet the goals; inhibiting irrelevant behaviors; and monitoring, regulating, and evaluating one's behaviors (Singer & Bashir, 1999; Ylvisaker & Feeney, 1995; Ylvisaker & Szekeres, 1989). The communicative consequences of disordered executive function include impaired topic maintenance, characterized by rambling or tangential utterances; vague referencing; dysfluent production; disinhibited and sometimes socially inappropriate utterances; hyperverbosity or restricted output; ineffectual verbal reasoning; and word-finding difficulties (Biddle, McCabe, & Bliss, 1996; Ylvisaker, 1992). In addition, individuals with TBI may also show confabulation by exaggerating events (Blosser & dePompei, 1989). Cultural, personality, and experiential variables also influence executive functioning (Ylvisaker & DuBonis, 2000).

Communication and executive function have reciprocal influences on each other (Ylvisaker & Feeney, 1995). Appropriate communication is needed for effective executive functioning. For example, the ability to communicate in a self-talk manner facilitates the regulation of behavior, which is an executive function (Singer & Bashir, 1999). Similarly, intact executive function is required for effective communication. For example, the ability to plan and organize one's thoughts is required to produce a coherent message. The interaction of communication and executive function is critical in understanding the functioning of individuals with TBI.

Assessment Applications

1. Tests of acquired aphasia or syntax are not applicable for individuals with TBI (Biddle, McCabe, & Bliss, 1996). The areas of deficit—communication and cognition—will not be adequately covered in these measures.

2. Clinicians need to assess cognitive functioning as well as discourse. Abilities in organization, planning, problem solving, and metacognition should be assessed.

3. Motivational and other factors (e.g., personality, home influences, and peer relationships) should also be assessed because they influence intervention.

Intervention Applications

1. Intervention needs to include the metacognitive skill of self-monitoring (Singer & Bashir, 1999).

2. Intervention cannot be decontextualized; real-life contexts need to be used, such as going to a restaurant or movies, attending social events, handling money, and employment settings (Singer & Bashir, 1999; Ylvisaker & DuBonis, 2000).

3. Language should be employed to guide, organize, and regulate behavior (Singer & Bashir, 1999). For example, speakers need to be able to use language to plan events (e.g., trips and parties) and monitor their behavior (e.g., use language to modify their responses if they are off target or tangential).

Introduction to the Sample

Leslie was enrolled in an outpatient remedial rehabilitation program, specializing in traumatic brain injury. She sustained her injury one year before the sample was elicited.

Leslie

10 years, 4 months

Leslie: 1. I'm going out with my mom today.

C: Oh, and you're going to do what?

L: 2. Do some house work today.

C: House work? What kind of housework are you going to do?

L: 3. No, I did housework today.

C: What did you do?

L: 4. And you know what?

C: What?

L: 5. I made some, um, uh, a little cotton ball and I stick it somewhere and 6. I made something for my mom and my grandma.

C: Oh did they like it?

L: 7. My other school, I did it.

C: That's really good. So how long is your grandma going to stay with you?

L: 8. Um, two weeks.

C: And then is she going back to Scotland?

L: 9. Yeah, no, she going sit there half an hour. 10. Half an hour she going to leave. 11. No, she gonna stay in my house at, um, 10:30.

C: Oh.

L: 12. No, she gonna leave here, not gonna leave. 13. She gonna stay here.

C: She's gonna stay?

L: 14. Yeah she is. 15. And I get her a bed, uh sleep with . . . 16. I get her a bed. 17. I made her a bed.

C: Does she sleep in your room?

L: 18. No.

C: In another room by herself?

L: 19. Yeah, Uncle Robert, um, Uncle Robert sleeps in a blue room.

C: In the blue room?

L: 20. Yeah with my dad . . . . . 21. My mom got mad at me. 22. She mad at me because I won't do my bedroom.

C: You won't clean your bedroom?

L: 23. No, last night I woke my mommy and my daddy up. 24. Guess what? 25. I'm mad at my mom.

C: Why are you mad at her?

L: 26. Because, um, no she not mad at me because um, because I won't do my bedroom.

C: Why won't you do your bedroom?

L: 27. She mad at me because she yelling at me at lunch time.

C: Is she mad because you didn't clean your bedroom?

L: 28. No.

C: Why is she mad at you?

L: 29. I did my bedroom a lot.

C: That's good.

L: 30. My parents went uh banquet.

C: They went where?

L: 31. A banquet. 32. You know what a banquet is?

C: No.

L: 33. It's a little courses and she takes um little she go dance, like she has a dance. 34. It's a little dance and she go to . . . 35. And then Louie Picklehead said to me, "Are you going to get marry?" 36. And I said, "No." 37. My mom, my daddy, my dad came in and he he got all drunk 38. and I said, "Now, why are you doing that?" 39. He up early last night because he snore.

C: Loudly?

L: 40. Yeah, because, um you know why?

C: Why?

L: 41. Because I woke him up and he woke. 42. I won't . . . he won't go to school and he can't go to work because he late for work.

Questions

1. The contradictions in some of Leslie's utterances appear to reflect a difficulty with the self-monitoring aspect of impaired executive function. If Leslie monitored her utterances, she would be able to detect and correct contradictions in her production. Where do contradictions occur in Leslie's utterances?

2. Leslie's concreteness is evident in her reduced semantic development. For example, she does not completely understand and produce causality concepts expressed with *because*. What utterances are characterized by impaired comprehension and/or production of causality (note in 22 that her use of causality is appropriate)?

3. Leslie's impulsivity and lack of attention span are evident in her abrupt changes of topic. She cannot disinhibit her impulses, so she talks about whatever comes to mind without making transitions. Usually the new topics are related by associations to the former topics. Where do you notice abrupt changes of topics?

4. What would be your intervention goals (consider both executive function and communicative effectiveness) for Leslie?

5. Describe a task that would incorporate the goals of improving both executive function and communication. Show how both aspects would be involved in an intervention task.

Part Three

Cultural and Linguistic Diversity

The number of individuals from culturally and linguistically diverse communities continues to grow. Also, the number of individuals from multicultural and linguistic backgrounds, who are served by speech-language pathologists, has increased. Multicultural clients comprise 25 percent of the monthly caseload reported by speech-language pathologists (Janota, 1997). The largest proportion is African American, followed by individuals whose second language is English.

Clinicians need to distinguish a difference in language behavior that represents a dialect from a disorder that represents a language deficit. They also need to contrast limited English proficiency and a language disorder. These are significant challenges for speech-language pathologists (Montgomery, 1999).

Assessing language use of children from diverse cultures requires appreciation of the linguistic and communicative features of their community as well as of their cultural values. Children may be misdiagnosed as language impaired when the linguistic and communicative patterns of their community differ from those of their clinicians and teachers. Nonbiased

assessment procedures need to be implemented in order to prevent misdiagnoses of language impairment and to achieve valid assessments.

These issues will be raised in Chapter 13 with regard to African American English and in Chapter 14 with regard to Spanish-influenced English. Asian English was not used because of the variability among Asian languages and the paucity of samples from children with language impairments. I have worked with two consultants for these chapters. Professor Linda Bland-Stewart provided me with assistance regarding African American English. She has conducted research studying the linguistic features of African American English (Seymour, Bland-Stewart, & Green, 1998). She has read this chapter and has made contributions to its contents. Professor Adelaida Restrepo has also offered her expertise in Chapter 14, concerning Spanish and English usage. She has conducted research in bilingualism (see Restrepo, 1998). She has read and reread drafts of this chapter. I am grateful to these two individuals for their assistance in this section.

13

Dialect

African American English

African American English (AAE) is a rule-governed linguistic and communicative system that is spoken by many African American speakers in the United States (Washington, 1996). It encompasses the domains of syntax, phonology, morphology, and pragmatics. AAE is generally considered to be a dialect of Standard American English (SAE) although it has its own unique history and rules (Washington & Craig, 1944). It has a well-defined structure and should never be considered to reflect an impoverished form of SAE or a disorder.

AAE is influenced by many factors, such as gender (more boys than girls in preschool populations), educational level (more use with speakers of less education than more education), geographic location (predominance in urban areas and the South), socioeconomic level (more use at lower socioeconomic status levels), task (increased use with pictures than in free play), social situations (increased use in more informal than formal contexts), and linguistic complexity (increased use with complex sentences) (Craig & Washington, 1994, 1995; Terrell & Terrell, 1993; Washington, Craig, & Kushman, 1998). Some predominant features of AAE are variable use of the copula and auxiliary; optional use of inflections; *be* to signal habitual meaning; triple negation; *done* as an indication of past action; and similar word order for direct and indirect questions (Craig & Washington, 1994; Labov, 1972; Smitherman, 1977; 1983; Washington & Craig, 1994; Wolfram, 1986).

Some of these features reflect phonological influences. For example, final inflections may be absent in words that are characterized by final consonant clusters. Consonant clusters reduce at the ends of words (e.g., *desk→des*). When an *–ed* inflection is added to a word that ends in a consonant, the resultant final cluster may be reduced (*talked→talk*) (Seymour &

Roeper, 1999). Phonological features of AAE always co-occur with syntactic features of AAE (Bland-Stewart, 2000).

Some of the features of AAE are also signs of language impairment (Seymour, Bland-Stewart, & Green, 1998). The syntax of children with language impairment is frequently characterized by absence of the copula (also known as zero-copula), auxiliary, and inflections (Bliss, 1989; Leonard, 1998; Rice, 1994).

Clinicians and educators need to determine whether a child who uses AAE demonstrates typical language behavior or impaired language development. Frequently test data are used to assist clinicians in the identification of language disorders. However, the use of standardized tests with children from diverse cultural and linguistic backgrounds is inappropriate because few are standardized on appropriate populations (Campbell, 1996; Taylor, 1985; Vaughn-Cooke, 1983; Washington, 1996; Washington & Craig, 1992). A test is valid only if it has been constructed with appropriate content and incorporates suitable normative data (Taylor, 1985; Terrell, Battle, & Granthan, 1998; Van Keulen, Weddington, & DeBose, 1998; Vaughn-Cooke, 1983). Clinicians must be very cautious if they use a test; there are many examples of African American children with appropriate communicative skills who have not performed well on tests that have not been standardized appropriately.

An alternative to standardized testing is analysis of discourse samples. They may reflect nonbiased assessment procedures if they take into account the linguistic and communicative features of a child's community. For example, The BESS (Black English Sentence Scoring) procedure was designed to encompass AAE syntactic features (Nelson, 1998; Nelson & Hyter, 1990). When analyzing discourse, clinicians need to consider that membership in a culture does not necessarily mean that a speaker uses the linguistic features of the community. They should also realize that AAE usage is not an all-or-none phenomenon (Labov, 1972). Speakers who use AAE also use Standard American English (SAE). Variability among AAE and SAE is evident in the discourse of preschool children (Bliss & Allen, 1981; Washington & Craig, 1994; Wyatt, 1966).

A thorough language sample analysis is necessary to distinguish between difference and disorder. The following three approaches have been suggested:

1. *Distinction between noncontrastive and contrastive features* (Seymour, Bland-Stewart, & Green, 1998). A noncontrastive feature is present in both SAE and AAE (Seymour, Bland-Stewart, & Green, 1998). Examples consist of articles, complex sentences, conjunctions, demonstratives, modals, negatives, verb particles, prepositions, and grammatical pronouns (Seymour, Bland-Stewart, & Green, 1998). In the utterance, S*he should put that pen in the desk,* there are noncontrastive features of a pronoun (*she*), modal (*should*), demonstrative (*that*), and preposition (*in*). These forms are expected to be present in both SAE and AAE. Alternatively, a contrastive feature is present in AAE and not SAE. Examples include variable use of copulas and auxiliaries as well as frequent absence of the inflections of third-person singular (*s*), past *ed*, plural (*s*) and possessive (*s*) (Seymour, Bland-Stewart, & Green, 1998). An example is in the utterance, *She mad.* In this utterance, there is zero copula. This construction could be found in a speaker of AAE and a child with a language impairment (LI) (Seymour, Bland-Stewart & Green, 1998).

African American children with LI generally use fewer noncontrastive features than their peers with typical language development (TLD) (Seymour, Bland-Stewart, & Green, 1998). Clinicians should focus on noncontrastive features used by an AAE-speaking African American child (Seymour, Bland-Stewart, & Green, 1998).

There is variability within the category of contrastive features. An example is with the use of copulas and auxiliaries. African American children do not always use *is* and *are* forms (Seymour, Abdulkarim, & Johnson, 1999; Seymour, Bland-Stewart, Green, 1998). However, *was*, *were*, and *am* are generally used (Seymour, Abdulkarim, & Johnson, 1999). Zero copula might suggest a language impairment (Seymour, Abdulkarim, & Johnson, 1999). Another example of variability is the use of the copula following a pronoun or noun. A child who does not use the copula after a pronoun (e.g., *He late*) and uses it after a noun (e.g., *John is late*) is following the rules for AAE (Seymour, Bland-Stewart, Green, 1998). The copula is also expected in the utterance final position (e.g. *Yes he is*). A child who does not use the copula in any linguistic context is not following AAE rules. This child, upon further study, may be language impaired.

2. *Clause length and occurrence of complex sentences.* This analysis will also distinguish typical and impaired language development (Craig & Washington, 1994, 2000; Craig, Washington, & Thompson-Porter, 1998). These two linguistic features are relatively independent of AAE usage. Preschool and school-age children who have reduced clause length and limited complex sentence production would be suspected of exhibiting a language impairment (Craig & Washington, 1994, 2000; Craig, Washington, & Thompson-Porter, 1998).

3. *Criterion-referenced procedures.* These procedures are made by clinicians to study a specific feature of language behavior (Lund & Duchan, 1993). They are useful for the identification of language impairments. Stockman (1996) described a minimal competency core approach. A child needs to demonstrate basic knowledge in core areas in order to be considered to exhibit typical language development. Stockman identified core competencies in the areas of phonology, pragmatics, semantics, syntax, and morphosyntax.

Assessment Applications

1. A language sample analysis should be used to augment standardized test data. Standardized tests may not be valid for speakers of AAE.

2. Families and community members may need to be consulted in order to achieve a valid diagnosis of language impairment.

3. Assessment needs to take place in a variety of contexts and with a variety of conversational partners (e.g., in formal and informal speaking contexts, with partners who speak AAE and SAE, and with peers and adults).

4. Variability in usage must be assessed in different linguistic contexts.

Intervention Applications

The following recommendations for intervention have been offered (Campbell 1993; 1994, 1996; Seymour, Abdulkarim, & Johnson, 1999; Wyatt, 1997):

1. Clinicians should focus on treating a disorder and not a dialect.

2. Intervention targets should be based upon the expectations and communicative values of a child's culture.

3. Intervention goals should focus on improving communicative functioning. AAE should be preserved.

Introduction to Samples

In these samples, the children use AAE to varying extents. In the first sample, Will is a 3-year-old African American child with typical language development. There is no history of speech, language, or cognitive deficits; he is performing similarly to his peers.

In the second sample in this section, Richard is a 5-year-old child with a language disorder who uses AAE. His language disorder was identified from parental reports of limited communication and from a language sample analysis. He has experienced difficulties in sound and letter recognition. He has been enrolled in an intervention program for 6 months.

The third sample was produced by BJ, who is a 7-year-old child. He is enrolled in an oral program for children with severe hearing impairments. With aids, his right and left ear average 50 dB (500), 50 dB (1000), and 55 dB (2000).

Typical Language Development

Will
3 years, 0 months

Adult: Hi William! I saw Calida [his neighbor] today.

William: 1. Calida was at the cleaners'?

A: Yes her mommy brought her.

W: 2. Did she go to grandmother's house?

A: No, she was just there for a little while.

W: 3. I saw her at school.

A: I missed you when you were gone on vacation. What did you see?

W: 4. I saw some puppies down south.

A: What did you do with them?

W: 5. I hold them. 6. I pinch them.

A: Why did you pinch them?

W: 7. They were soft. 8. What this [points to a toaster oven]?

A: That's an oven.

W: 9. What do you do with it?

A: You cook food in it.

W: 10. You put something in it?

A: Yes. I like to cook. You don't cook, do you?

W: 11. I'm too little to cook.

A: Yes, I guess you are. How did you hurt yourself at school today?

W: 12. I ran to Erica.

A: Then what?

W: 13. Bump my nose on her. 14. She was playing on that pole.

A: Did you cry?

W: 15. I was crying! 16. It was bleeding. 17. It was all red.

A: Are you mad at her?

W: 18. I'm not gonna give her no more candy!

A: Did Mrs F help you?

W: 19. I'm not in Mrs F's room no more. 20. She in Room 6. 21. My momma bought you those [points to the adult's jeans].

A: No she didn't. I did.

W: 22. I gonna buy all the jeans [knocks his juice over].

A: Oh, what happened?

W: 23. It spill on my fingers.

A: I'll clean it up for you.

W: 24. Hey, where your bike at [points to a bike in the corner]?

A: It's at home.

W: 25. My daddy got one of those.

A: Here's a Tootsie Roll for you.

W: 26. It look like sausage. 27. It taste good.

A: I knew you would like it.

W: 28. Where Basil [adult's husband] at?

A: He's at home.

W: 29. He coming over here?

A: Not tonight, maybe tomorrow.

W: 30. Now we all finish [talking].

Language Impairment

Richard
5 years, 4 months

Adult: What do we have do with these blocks first?

Richard: 1. Put they back.

A: OK.

R: 2. That it? 3. Is there more there?

A: No.

R: 4. What this [wind-up toy] do?

A: You wind him up and he walks.

R: 5. How do it? [adult winds up the toy] 6. What him [he points to the toy] do?

A: He's walking.

R: 7. Why him tail moving?

A: I don't know. Is it moving when he walks?

R: 8. Uhuh, what them ?

A: Cards.

R: 9. What that? 10. What this?

A: It's a mat for some cars.

R: 11. Don't put they [cars] here [on the mat].

A: OK.

R: 12. Look, me have car. 13. Where . . . what . . . what one you gonna have?

A: I don't know. Which one do you want?

R: 14. This be mine. 15. That be yours.

A: OK.

R: 16. Open car. 17. How you open it?

A: I don't think that car opens.

R: 18. This open? [Batmobile]

A: Not really. What do you want to be, Batman or Robin?

R: 19. I be Batman. 20. We . . . you be Robin. 21. Robin, where you at?

A: I'm at the ice cream store. Where are you?

R: 22. I be home.

A: Can I come to your house? What should we do?

R: 23. We . . . we . . . we gonna sleep.

A: Sleep? That does not sound like much fun. I'm going now. Where should we go?

R: 24. I go my house. 25. Go back my home.

A: OK. We'll go to your house. How are you going to get there?

R: 26. I, I not taking car. 27. I taking Jeep. 28. Gimme Jeep.

A: I wonder if Batman goes to school.

R: 29. I gonna school.

A: What kinds of things happen at school?

R: 30. Your car coming? 31. Take him school [plays with cars and objects]. 32. Batman car can't go.

Hearing Impairment

BJ
7 years, 5 months

Adult: What did you do for spring break?

BJ: 1. Play.

A: What did you play with?

BJ: 2. Play floor.

A: What else did you do?

BJ: 3. Eat cookie. 4. I play outside.

A: What did you do outside?

BJ: 5. My bike.

A: Did you ride your bike?

BJ: 6. They push me. 7. I ride . . . I ride . . . I ride my . . . I ride by myself on the street.

A: Did you do anything else?

BJ: 8. Play with brother.

A: What did you do with your brother?

BJ: 9. He cry too much.

A: He cries too much?

BJ: 10. Yeah, he don't wanna play with me. 11. I too small. 12. I have baby. 13. My baby.

A: Your baby?

BJ: 14. No, not my baby.

A: Whose baby is it?

BJ: 15. Somebody let us have it.

A: Whose baby?

BJ: 16. Some . . . it somebody baby. 17. Her let us have it.

A: How long have you had the baby?

BJ: 18. Nine.

A: How <u>long</u> have you had the baby?

BJ: 19. No, he like . . . he know how eat crackers.

A: The baby?

BJ: 20. But . . . but . . . but he . . . but he . . . know how grab something.

A: Really?

BJ: 21. He one year. 22. He bite. 23. He got two teeth right here [points to his bottom jaw].

A: That's nice. What do you do with him?

BJ: 24. He . . . he . . . he cry if . . . if he bump his head. 25. He gonna cry.

A: What do you do for him?

BJ: 26. Just get him out the floor. 27. Lay him on, on, on pillow and put bottle on him.

A: I bet he likes that.

BJ: 28. He don't like bump head. 29. If I were doing like this, [gestures how the baby bumps his head] he don't wanna bump his head. 30. He always bump his head.

A: Why?

BJ: 31. On basket. 32. He playing. 33. He bump his head. 34. He cried. 35. Me, me, I hafta get him up. 36. He climb on chair.

Questions (for Will's sample)

1. Identify utterances that have the following <u>contrastive features</u>:

Copula

    present:

    absent:

Auxiliary

    present:

    absent:

Plural *s*

    present:

    absent:

Past *ed*

    present:

    absent:

Possessive *s*

    present:

    absent:

Third-person singular *s*

    present:

    absent:

2. Identify the utterances that have the following <u>noncontrastive</u> features:

Articles

    present:

    absent:

Pronouns: Just look at subject pronouns (*I, she, he,* and *they*) and identify only four occurrences.

grammatical use:

substitutions:

Prepositions (*at, to, in and on*)

present:

absent:

Complex sentences

present:

3. Does analysis of contrastive versus noncontrastive features support the fact that Will has typical language development, in your opinion? Why or why not?

4. Does Will use both SAE and AAE features? Support your answer.

5. According to Seymour, Abdulkarim, and Johnson (1999), children who use AAE generally omit *is* and *are* and use *am, was,* and *were.* Does this statement reflect Will's usage?

Is/are

present:

absent:

Am/was/were

present:

absent:

Questions (for Richard's sample)

1. Identify the utterances that are characterized by the presence or absence of the following contrastive features:

Auxiliaries

    present:

    absent:

Copulas (*is/are*)

    present:

    absent:

Possessive *s*

    present:

    absent:

There were no obligatory contexts for plural, past, and third-person singular forms.

2. Identify the utterances that are characterized by the presence and absence of the following noncontrastive features:

Articles

    present:

    absent:

Pronouns

    grammatical subject *I* pronoun:

    ungrammatical subject pronouns:

    ungrammatical object pronouns:

    ungrammatical possessive pronouns:

Prepositions

present:

absent:

Complex sentences

present:

Other: Does Richard use adjectives either before or after nouns? If so, where?

3. Richard uses the word *be*, which is used by speakers of AAE to convey a habitual meaning, somewhat similar to the meaning of *always* in SAE. It is used to convey repeated activity and is more powerful than *always*. (a) Where does he use this form? (b) Does Richard use it to convey a habitual meaning? (c)Why could he be using this form?

4. Does the analysis of noncontrastive versus contrastive feature use support the finding that Richard has a language impairment? Support your answer.

5. Compare Will and Richard with respect to contrastive and noncontrastive features.

6. What intervention goals would you identify for Richard?

Questions (for BJ's sample)

1. Identify the utterances that are characterized by the presence or absence of the following contrastive features:

Auxiliaries

    present:

    absent:

Copulas

    present:

    absent:

Plural *s*

    present:

    absent:

Past *ed*

    present:

    absent:

Possessive *s*

    present:

    absent:

Third-person singular *s*

    present:

    absent:

2. Identify the utterances that are characterized by the presence or absence of the following noncontrastive features:

Articles

   present:

   absent:

Pronouns

   grammatical use of subject pronouns (*I, he, they*) <u>Only give four examples</u>:

   substitution of subject pronouns:

Prepositions

   present:

   absent:

   substitution:

Complex sentences

   present (include ungrammatical attempts):

3. There are features of language impairment in BJ's sample. Discuss his behavior with respect to the following:

Response to questions:

   Appropriate semantic contingency in his answers to questions (what responses answer the questions that were asked?):

   What answers are reduced in semantic contingency?

   Dysfluencies:

      Pauses:

      Repetitions:

      Internal corrections:

4. Does the analysis of contrastive versus noncontrastive feature use in BJ's sample suggest a language impairment? Support your answer.

5. Does BJ show knowledge of both SAE and AAE? Why?

6. Contrast Richard and BJ with respect to their language usage (contrastive and noncontrastive features as well as other aspects of their language use).

7. What intervention goals would you identify for BJ?

14

Bilingualism

Spanish-Influenced English

Before I begin this chapter, I want to describe my background with respect to bilingualism. I am a monolingual speech-language pathologist who has recently moved to an area of the United States in which many children from Mexican American families live. In my recent research, I arranged to have discourse samples collected from Spanish-speaking children with typical and impaired language development. Spanish-speaking students elicited the samples in both English and Spanish. Bilingual speakers, both students and professionals, helped analyze and interpret the discourse. Many times my lack of knowledge of Spanish resulted in erroneous interpretations of some utterances. For example, there were utterances that I thought reflected unusual constructions in English. According to my bilingual collaborators, the speaker was translating from Spanish into English (e.g., *We stay on the night.*). My research pointed out the complexity of the field of bilingualism. In this chapter, some of the pertinent issues in this area are introduced. I recommend that you extend your reading beyond this chapter (see Kayser, 1998b; Kayser & Restrepo, 1995).

Nature of bilingualism. Bilingualism is the ability to speak two languages. The bilingual (and multilingual) population in the United States is growing every year (U.S. Bureau of the Census, 1996). Bilingualism represents a range of abilities in both languages (Kayser, 1998b). Linguistic proficiency can vary in each language depending upon the contexts in which each language is used. Speech-language pathologists need to differentiate a language disorder from reduced knowledge of English.

Individuals learn two (or more) languages differently, depending upon their experiences at home and at school. Some children learn two or more languages simultaneously before they are 3 years old (Kayser,

1998b). This pattern of simultaneous language acquisition is most prevalent when a child is exposed to different languages in the home, with an emphasis on one language. Another pattern of bilingualism is the acquisition of one language in the home and the acquisition of a second language at school after the age of 3 years (Kayser, 1998b). This pattern of successive acquisition occurs more frequently in bilingualism. Simultaneous acquisition is generally associated with a more equal ability to use both languages than successive acquisition.

Age of acquisition and motivational, contextual (e.g., language spoken in the home), and societal (e.g., status of the first language) factors influence second-language learning (Kayser, 1998b). Moreover, clinicians need to understand when and how children learn both languages (Peña & Jackson, 2000). Awareness of the circumstances in which children become bilingual will help the clinician make appropriate clinical judgments about their language learning abilities (Gutiérrez-Clellen et al., 2000; Peña & Jackson, 2000).

Contextual factors influence linguistic performance in both languages (Gutiérrez-Clellen et al., 2000). For example, the contexts of home and school may show variations in language use. Children may have knowledge of specific words that are used at home (e.g., regarding social functions, religion, and food) in their first language (L-1) and may show a different lexical knowledge in their second language (L-2), such as words frequently used in school (e.g., for colors and numbers) (Gutiérrez-Clellen et al., 2000; Kayser, 1998a).

Code switching is a communicative style that is commonly used by bilingual speakers (Kayser, 1995a). It is characterized by the insertion of a word or phrase in a language that is different from the one that is used. It is often used to quote someone, emphasize a point, or express a concept or word that does not have a translation in the other language (Grossjean, 1982). It serves to assist a speaker in communicating ideas and does not generally represent an impairment (Kayser, 1995a). An example of code switching was provided by Tatiana, a 5-year-old child with typical language development. She was talking in English to a bilingual Spanish-speaking adult. She inserted the word *bruja* (witch) and the phrase *la mamma de Gavi* (Gavi's mother) in her discourse. In the first instance, she may not have known the English word. In the second occurrence, she may have used an expression that she has frequently heard in Spanish. Tatiana was aware that the listener knew Spanish and the identity of Gavi; she used code switching to augment her message. However, code switching may also be a sign of a possible problem when a speaker uses another language with which the listener is unfamiliar. In this instance, the speaker does not realize that the listener cannot understand the insertion. Code switching may also reflect limited knowledge in the second language (Gutiérrez-Clellen, 1996).

Spanish-influenced English (SiE). In this chapter, the bilingualism of Spanish and English is highlighted in successive language acquisition. Spanish was selected because of the growing number of Spanish speakers in the United States (U.S. Bureau of the Census, 1996). The number of Spanish speakers is expected to grow from 31 million to 63 million between 2000 and 2030 (U.S. Bureau of the Census, 1996).

Children who speak Spanish as a first language come from a variety of cultural and linguistic backgrounds, such as Mexico, Puerto Rico, Cuba, and Central and South America. Mexican American groups represent the largest percentage of Spanish speakers in the United States (Kayser, 1998b). Although the term, "Spanish" is used to describe the language that may be spoken in these areas, there is variation in the Spanish that is used among and within different countries (Gutiérrez-Clellen, 1996; Kayser, 1989). Thus, variability should be expected among speakers of different dialects of Spanish (Gutiérrez-Clellen, 1996; Kayser, 1995b). There is also variability in the acquisition of a first and subsequent languages (Anderson, 1994; Gutiérrez-Clellen, 1999). Children who are learning to speak Spanish and English may use a combination of both rules in their language usage (Kayser & Restrepo, 1995).

Children who come from Spanish-speaking homes and who are learning English as a second language may use SiE (Kayser, 1989; Langdon, 1992). SiE is English that has been influenced by Spanish forms. Some features of SiE are (Anderson, 1996; Kayser, 1989, 1989 1998b; Kayser & Restrepo, 1995; Langdon, 1989):

Absence of inflections, articles, the *do* and other auxiliaries, and copulas.

Definite article used frequently in contexts that are not common in English (e.g., *I washed the hand*).

Subject pronouns may be absent if they have been previously identified.

Present tense used for irregular past-tense verbs (e.g., *come* for *came*).

Prepositions may be omitted or substituted (in Spanish, location is not emphasized as frequently as in English).

Subject-verb nonagreement (e.g., *She have money*).

No used for *not* in sentences and *no* for *don't* in imperatives.

Adjectives may be used after the noun (e.g., *cat gray*).

Use of simple sentences.

Clinical implications of bilingualism. Some features that have been considered to be indications of a language disorder in monolingual speakers cannot be considered to be signs of language impairment in some bilingual speakers. For example, word revisions, latency in responding, and frequent pauses between words may not indicate a language disorder for bilingual speakers (Gutiérrez-Clellen, 1996). They may be produced while a speaker searches for appropriate words in the second language (L-2). Dysfluencies could reflect cultural and stylist variations evident in L-1 and may be evident in specific contexts and not in others. For example, there may be situations in which a speaker is not prepared to use the second language (L-2) but is asked to do so, as in school where only English is used. The child's production may be halting because of the unexpected speaking requirements of the situation. Other linguistic features that are not parallel in monolingual and bilingual usage are the use of concrete vocabulary and simple sentences. In monolingual school-aged children they may be signs of a language impairment. In bilingual children these features may reflect a communicative strategy that is used to avoid difficult forms in order to facilitate communication (Kayser, 1998b).

In Spanish, the following measures were found to predict language impairment: parental report of speech and language skills, increased grammatical errors per T-Unit (similar to a clause), reduced T-Unit length, and family history of speech and language problems (Restrepo, 1998). These features are also common features of language impairment in English speakers (Nelson, 1998; Paul, 2001).

The diagnosis of language impairment must be made in both languages (Anderson, 1996; Kayser, 1995b). A monolingual clinician needs to refer a child to a bilingual speech-language pathologist for an appropriate diagnosis. A Spanish-speaking child with a language disorder will show a disorder in L-1 and L-2. The disorder can be manifested differently in both languages, depending on the linguistic characteristics of each. If there are limitations only in L-2, the child would appear to be having difficulty learning English and would have limited English proficiency and not a language impairment.

Assessment Applications

1. Bilingual speech-language pathologists need to make the diagnosis of language disorder. Both L-1 and L-2 need to be assessed in a variety of contexts and with different conversational partners.

2. Members of the child's family and community as well as teachers should be consulted in order to determine the language history, proficiency and experiences of a child (Gutiérrez-Clellen et al., 2000; Pearson, Fernández, & Oller, 1993). The amount and age of exposure to English at home and at school need to be determined. The profi-

ciency of language use in different contexts should also be explored.

3. Test data should be interpreted cautiously, if at all, unless there are well-developed norms that have been derived from the child's culture.

Intervention Applications

1. Intervention should be implemented in both languages.

2. The clinician should include in intervention culturally relevant material, such as literature, food, and holidays (Kayser, 1995a).

3. Consultations with bilingual professionals and use of paraprofessionals will aid the clinician.

Introduction to the Samples

The samples in this section were elicited from children who come from Mexican American backgrounds. Their first language, Spanish, is spoken at home. They learned English when they began school at 5 years of age. They speak English in school and are receiving education in English.

Juan and David have been diagnosed as language impaired by a bilingual speech-language pathologist. They scored below the mean for their chronological ages on two language tests, one in English and one in Spanish. Both their teachers and parents reported that they encountered difficulty in communicating in both Spanish and English. According to David's mother, he is dysfluent in both languages.

Goals for intervention will not be addressed in this section because the language samples elicited in Spanish are not available and many of the readers (including me) are not bilingual. Goals for intervention need to be identified on the basis of the quality of language samples in both Spanish and English.

Typical Language Development

Jose
9 years

Adult: I heard you were in a fight. What happened?

Jose: 1. I fight with my friend because he was not playing well.

A: What did you do about it?

J: 2. I fights with him 3. and he fight back to me.

A: Did you get into trouble?

J: 4. Then we get out. 5. Then my mom called and called me and hit me because I was being bad.

A: What happened to your friend?

J: 6. My friend cry. 7. I bleed him and blind him. 8. Then he went to his mom 9. and then his mom come, came on our house 10. and and she tell that I was fighting with him.

A: What did your mom say?

J: 11. My mom said that I was bad. 12. I said that I know that.

Language Impairment

Juan
6 years, 9 months

A: Have you ever had a bee sting? [child nods] Tell me about it.

J: 1. [points to his eye] On my eye. 2. Me got a bee sting.

A: I can see it's red.

J: 3. I go to the doctor. 4. Me go to sleep all the times . . . night time. 5. and that finish and finish and getting little and little and little . . . 6. My eye close and close all the time and 7. and me put some ice and 8. it was open and open.

A: It got all better?

J: 9. [nods yes] And one time, me see on the mirror, it's no more!

A: Where were the bees?

J: 10. On the water . . . them crawlin'. 11. Them go buzz . . . 12. and them hit us on the . . . [points to head].

A: Did they hurt you?

J: 13. mhhhm . . . .Sting. 14. Them got fat and fat.

A: The bees stings got fat? That hurts?

J: 15: We fishin' with my dad.

A: Who else was there?

J: 16: And my family.

A: And the bees were in the water?

J: 17. Yeah, and the bugs.

A: Bugs too?

J: 18. mhhmm On the day, we stay on the night . . . with the coyotes. 19. and my brother . . . see . . . 20. When we go in the night to get some beer for my dad . . . we see some coyotes hiding and some wolf, like crawling and crawling [pantomimes] 21. and we take off!

A: Was it scary?

J: 22. Yeah and we jump the fence and we calling dad . . . 23. He he not . . . 24. Them not kill him 25. but them already gone and and go back home to eat fish.

A: Did you have fish for dinner?

J: 26. mhmm . . . My dad like 'em. 27. Me hate fish. 28. Them stinks! 29. Then me get a drink. 30. Me go to sleep.

Language Impairment

David
6 years, 0 months

Adult: I heard you were in the hospital. What happened to you?

David: 1. I was umm . . . 2. There was um a doctor because . . . there was some uh somebody in trouble. 3. They were in trouble.

A: Who was in trouble?

D: 4. Somebody.

A: What happened to him?

D: 5. Um . . . Danielle [listener did not know the identity of this person], she go to hospital . . . 6. and there was um . . . 7. There . . . 8. And and the hospital in trouble . . . um . . . um . . . 9. The man . . . 10. and there was some . . . 11. The hospital because . . . 12. There was um . . . 13. This hospital . . . 14. And the and the girl was sleepy 15. And the bed with his dad.

A: What happened to Danielle?

D: 16. Nothing.

A: What else happened at the hospital?

D: 17. Nothing.

Questions (for Jose's sample)

1. Where are there the following SiE features in Jose's discourse?

Present tense for irregular past-tense verbs:

Absence of inflections:

Substitutions of prepositions:

2. Jose also uses English versions of these and other non-SiE features. Show where.

Use of irregular verbs:

Use of the capula and auxiliary:

Use of inflections:

Use of subject pronouns:

3. Are there utterances that do not appear to represent SiE? They may reflect incomplete mastery of English, use of a child's unique rule system, or a language impairment. If so, identify these utterances.

Questions (for Juan's sample)

1. Where are there SiE features in Juan's discourse?

Present tense substituted for past tense:

Absence of inflections:

Absence of subject pronouns:

Absence of copulas and auxiliaries (including the perfective):

Substitutions of prepositions

2. Juan also uses English versions of these and other non-SiE features. Show where.

Use of subject pronouns (although they may be ungrammatical, the subject is present):

Use of inflections:

Use of irregular verbs:

Use of copulas:

3. Are there utterances that do not appear to represent SiE? They may reflect incomplete mastery of English use of a child's unique rule system or a language impairment. If so, identify these utterances.

4. What would be the reasons for enrolling Juan in an intervention program and what are the reasons against enrolling him?

Questions (for David's sample)

David's difficulties are with discourse coherence. He exhibits the same problems in Spanish as in English. He is unfamiliar with the adult who is eliciting the sample.

1. Show where David is dysfluent.

Abandoned utterances:

    Repetitions:

    Excessive pauses:

    Internal corrections:

    Fillers:

2. Where does he show inappropriate referencing?

3. What utterances cannot be clearly understood?

Part Four

Assessment

The purpose of Part Four is to consider issues that clinicians frequently encounter in assessment. Two issues focus on the representativeness of a sample and discourse variability. A clinician needs to determine whether the language behavior that was elicited in the clinic reflects a child's functional communication. A representative sample is critical for appropriate clinical decisions to be made. For example, if a child is relatively quiet, the clinician may think that the child exhibits an impairment. However, the child may speak freely with peers and family members. A representative sample may not always be possible to elicit because the clinical context is not typical of functional communication; it is structured and decontextualized. In order to obtain a representative sample the clinician needs to understand that discourse changes in different contexts.

Discourse changes with conversational participants who are familiar or unfamiliar (Sonnenschien,

1986) and who differ in age (Sachs & Devin, 1976; Shatz & Gelman, 1973). This variability occurs for speakers with both typical and impaired language development (Bliss, 1984; Fey & Leonard, 1984; Fey, Leonard, & Wilcox, 1981). The clinician needs to consider variability to determine whether a clinical sample is representative of a child's functional communication.

In Chapter 15, the differences between home and clinic samples are compared. In Chapter 16, variability between different discourse genres is explored. In Chapter 17, variability between test and test performance and spontaneous language behavior are studied. These chapters relate to the representativeness and variability of discourse. The final chapter, 18, focuses on many aspects of language and communicative function rather than studying separate behaviors, as has been done previously. Four language samples were elicited from children at different levels of language use.

15
Comparison of Home and Clinic Samples

A language sample that has been elicited in a clinical setting may not reflect a child's communicative functioning outside of this context. In a familiar context with known individuals, a child could use behaviors that are different from those that are elicited in a clinical context. Samples produced at home by mothers and in a clinic by clinicians are similar with respect to the number and diversity of words, semantic relations, and complex sentences (Kramer, James, & Saxman, 1979; Olswang & Carpenter, 1978). They also differ from each other in that mothers' elicitations contain more utterances and longer sentences than clinicians' samples (Kramer, James, & Saxman, 1979; Olswang & Carpenter, 1978).

In this chapter, two samples are compared, one elicited by a child's mother at home and one elicited by a student clinician. The student was familiar with the child.

Assessment Applications

1. Clinicians should elicit samples in more than one context (e.g., clinic, home, classroom, and recess) and with different conversational partners (e.g., parents and peers).
2. If a home sample cannot be obtained, a parent or teacher should be interviewed to determine how the child communicates outside of the clinical setting.

3. Samples should also be elicited, when possible, with a child's siblings to see how the discourse varies from that of the parents and the clinician.

Intervention Applications

1. Clinicians should use parents and other caregivers to assist the generalization of forms that have been targeted in intervention (Owens, 1999).
2. Some parents may be too demanding or busy to work with their children. However, if parents are used, they need to be systematically trained to help their child. Sending homework home without parental training is not generally helpful (Fey, 1986).
3. Intervention should be carried out in different contexts (e.g.,. classroom, recess, and home) to enhance generalization (Bliss, 1993; Owens, 1999).

Introduction to the Samples

Jeff is a 3-year-old child who has been receiving language remediation for 4 months. The clinician was familiar with Jeff; she had been working with him since he was enrolled in an intervention program.

Jeff
3 years, 5 months

Home Sample

Jeff: 1. Me turn light on. 2. Me don't turn lights out, mom. 3. Me turn lights on. 4. King's dog, "Woo-woo-woo." 5. Markie [his brother], "Woo-woo-woo."

Mother: You like your cereal?

J: 6. I don't like.

M: You don't like your cereal?

J: 7. Mark eat my cereal.

M: This is sugar pops.

J: 8. Mom, mine not.

M: This is the cereal I'm eating.

J: 9. Me eat Mark's cereal. 10. Eat Mark cereal. 11. Me eat Mark's cereal [J goes into the bedroom to dress].

M: Come on, fix your pants.

J: 12. No, no, me, me [wants to fix his pants himself].

M: What?

J: 13. Put down here? 14. Put down here [wants cereal to be taken off the counter].

M: All right. I'll put it down here, just a minute.

J: 15. Mom, put down here!

M: All right, but if I put it down there, Boo [their cat] will get it.

J: 16. No, put it down here, please. 17. Put it down here, Mom. 18. Put it down here. 19. Mom, watch. [looks at the tape recorder]. 20. Put up. 21. Put up, mom. 22. Put button. 23. Mom, push button.

M: No, we don't need to touch it right now. It is fine where it is.

J: 24. Me push. 25. Me do it [pointing to clothes that need to be folded]. 26. Me do mine [picks up a pair of pants and folds them in half]. 27. Mom, look!

M: That's good. Now fold it again.

J: 28. Make two?

M: Let's fold the pants. You know how to do that.

J: 29. Mark's pants. 30. Me do it now, ma . . . 31. Mark's pants.

M: Lay them out like this. Your pants are back there.

J: 32. Lay out, Mom. 33. Lay out.

M: Do you want to help me put these clothes away?

J: 34. No.

M: Somebody is at the door.

J: 35. Mark [goes to the door and returns to the kitchen]. 36. Mom, play cards. 37. Mark.

Clinic Sample

Clinician: What color is Tinkerbelle?

J: 38. Kitten.

C: Yes, she is a kitten, but what color is she? [Jeff does not respond] Tink is this big. Is Boo [his cat] bigger?

J: 39. No [gestures a size].

C: That big.

J: 40. No, big [enlarges the size].

C: Bigger?

J: 41. Big [enlarges the size again but appropriate for a cat].

C: Is Boo the biggest cat in your house?

J: 42. BIG! [arms outstretched and then he picks up a movable toy figure and starts to manipulate it]. 43. Look, sitting.

C: That's right. He's sitting.

J: 44. No, sitting. 45. Move head [Jeff rotates toy's head and puts the toy in different positions and describes what the toy is doing]. 46. Man walking. 47. Move head [Jeff rotates the toy's head]. 48. Man sit down. 49. Man lay down. 50. Man stand up. 51. Man sit down [reaches for the female doll]. 52. Lady walking.

C: Make the lady sit down.

J: 53. Sitting. 54. Move head [rotates the toy's head, reaches for a plastic lion and puts the animal in different positions and describes what the lion is doing]. 55. Lion standing. 56. Fall down [makes the lion fall down]. 57. Lion up [makes the lion stand]. 58. Lion standing. 59. Move head [rotates the lion's head]. 60. Lion fall down. 61. Lion stand.

C: What is this? [car]

J: 62. Car.

C: Yes, and what is the car doing? [moves the car]

J: 63. Car rolling.

C: Yes, the car is rolling.

J: 64. Car up, mom [rolls the car up his arm]. 65. Car off [takes car off his arm]. 66. Car turn [puts car on table and rolls it]. 67. Stop [the car stopped]. 68. Me feel OK. 69. Car up [puts car on his arm]. 70. Car roll down [makes car roll down his arm and then knocks over a pile of blocks].

Questions

1. You will compare Jeff's assertive conversational acts in both contexts. Compare the frequency and type (e.g., requests for information or requests for action) of Jeff's requests at home and in the clinic. Hint: Look at the preceding and following utterances to determine his communicative intent.

Home:

Requests for information:

Requests for action:

Clinic:

Requests for information:

Requests for action:

2. Compare the frequency and type (e.g., requests for information or requests for action) of requests produced by Jeff's mother and clinician.

Mother's requests (before which utterances):

Requests for information:

Requests for action:

Clinician's requests (before which utterances):

Requests for information:

Requests for action:

What is the difference between the quality of the questions asked by Jeff's mother and his clinician?

3. List the Agent + Action + Object structures that Jeff used at home and at the clinic.

Home:

Clinic:

4. What is the importance of the difference between the two contexts for assessment?

5. What are your intervention goals for Jeff?

16

Discourse Coherence
Genre Variability

Discourse coherence is discussed within the same framework that was presented in Chapter 6. The conversational rules presented by Grice (1975) describe coherence in discourse genres other than conversation, such as scripts (e.g., descriptions of routine events), procedural discourse (e.g., descriptions of procedures), narration or story telling, and expository discourse (e.g., explanation, argumentation, verbal problem solving). The conversational principles described by Grice (1975) are quantity (informativeness and referencing), quality (truth), relation (relevance or topic maintenance), and manner (fluency).

Discourse coherence varies among different genres. For example, dysfluencies are more evident in narratives than in conversations (MacLachlan & Chapman, 1988; Wagner, Nettelbladtt, Sahlen, & Nilhom, 2000). Narratives are associated with longer utterances than conversations (Leadholm & Miller, 1992). Differences in discourse coherence among genres are evident because some tasks are more difficult than others. Narratives and expository discourse impose burdens on a speaker that are not evident in conversation. Planning and organization are involved in these more advanced forms of discourse. A speaker needs to organize thoughts and sequence events more in narration and expository discourse than in conversation. As processing demands increase, dysfluencies are evident (Dollaghan & Campbell, 1992; Leadholm & Miller, 1992; MacLachlan & Chapman, 1988). In contrast, conversation is structured; the listener often controls the discourse by asking direct questions. This genre does not impose a burden on a speaker. Length is another influence on discourse coherence. Conversations usually involve shorter utterances than narratives and expository discourse. Referencing abilities of children with language impairment decrease with longer utterances (Purcell & Liles, 1992).

Discourse should be elicited in a variety of genres in order to determine if there is a disorder and where a communication breakdown occurs (Lahey, 1990). In a conversation, a child may not show impairments that are evident in more demanding genres, such as narration or expository discourse. Success in these genres is critical for academic achievement (McCabe & Rollins, 1994; Nelson, 1998). Assessment in challenging discourse genres is critical to determine potential for academic proficiency.

In this chapter, discourse variability will be examined in genres. In the first sample, the speaker described a routine at school (e.g., a script) and a unique form of a baseball game (e.g., expository or procedural discourse). In the second exercise, two other genres (conversation and narration) were elicited and will be compared.

Assessment Applications

1. Clinicians need to assess variability in discourse ability by examining a variety of discourse genres (e.g., conversation and narratives).

2. Elicitation of conversational discourse cannot be held as an interview, by bombarding a child with a series of questions. Samples should be elicited in relatively informal contexts, such as playing with objects.

3. Discourse coherence is maximized when a speaker is motivated to communicate new information (Hudson & Shaprio, 1991). Questions, therefore, should relate to experiences and events that are not known to the clinician.

Intervention Applications

1. Hierarchies in intervention can be developed from simple to more complex discourse forms, from those that involve minimal planning to those that involve considerable discourse planning.

2. Scripts and procedural discourse will be easier to elicit from most children than narratives and expository discourse (Bliss, 1993).

3. Within each genre there may be levels of complexity. For example, regarding procedural discourse, describing how to make a peanut butter and jelly sandwich is easier than describing how to play football (Bliss, 1993).

Introduction to the Samples

Alan sustained a traumatic brain injury when he was 11 years old. At the time of this sample, he lived in a residential school for children with severe learning disabilities and brain injury. He returned home on the weekends. The two samples in this example were edited from a 100-utterance sample. The remaining utterances consisted of brief responses to questions asked of Alan.

Robin is 8 years old. He has been diagnosed as language learning impaired with attention deficit hyperactivity disorder. He has been enrolled in special classes for children with language impairment since he was 4 years old.

Alan
12 years

Clinician: Do you have a **routine** that you have to do (in the residential home)?

Alan: 1. Have to do curtains.

C: Oh, those are your chores?

A: 2. We, we sometimes go outside and play [sounds like "pray"].

C: You pray?

A: 3. We <u>play</u> in the gym or outside 4. and we have breakfast and supper here. 5. We, we, we, have watch our TV and sit down and have orange or apple 6. and they give us half hour quiet time so quiet down 7. and . . . . that's it.

C: I heard you had a **baseball** game here last week but it was different. Why?

A: 8. Staff against children.

C: And you had some special rules, right?

A: 9. The guy that stays in the middle, he . . . 10. If the guy catch gets it, they have to go out 11. but if the guy hits the ball at the pitcher, he's out. 12. If he hits the pitcher and the other guy in the middle . . . 13. Like, if the ball pass him that way, he suppose to take one foot out of circle. 14. If he takes both out, he have home run. 15. That's it.

Robin
8 years

Conversation

Clinician: What are you going to do in Colorado?

Robin: 1. . . . A lot of stuff, go to the mountains, throw rocks at the sea . . . 2. It's warm there 3. 'cuz it's summer there too 4. but their only summer is only 14 weeks . . . in the summer.

C: Who is going?

R: 5. . . . My sister unless she doesn't want to go. 6. I don't want her to go.

C: Are you going by yourself?

R: 7. No . . . my dad's flying on a plane here 8. and then we're flying there.

C: So, you're flying to Colorado?

R: 9. Uh-huh [yes] . . . but we're gonna drive back.

C: Where are you getting the car?

R: 10. My dad rents one from his . . . his boss. 11. He's got all these . . . RVs. 12. Last time when we went, we drove back. 13. We drove over to Colorado 14. and we flew back 15. but this time we're flying there and then back.

Personal Narrative

C: Did your sister ever have to go to the hospital? [nods yes]. What happened?

R: 16. She broke legs 17. and uh a dog bit her right here [points to leg] 18. and it went through her knee.

C: What happened?

R: 19. Um . . . my my mom was taking care of this dog. 20. It used to be nice 21. and she she didn't know it was still nice 22. and that and that she did that 23. and the dog like bit her. 24. The dog was uh mad 25. and then and then my mom uh my mom my mom did something like . . . 26. don't know. 27. I forgot. 28. I forgot what she did. 29. She like hit the dog.

C: She hit the dog?

R: 30. Yeah, put some water on it.

C: She did? Then what?

R: 31. Well . . . that was it 32. and then and then and then she went to the hospital 33. and it was . . . 34. When she was going, both of the doors opened.

C: Both of the doors?

R: 35. Yeah in the back. 36. She was lying down 37. and then both of the doors opened. 38. That's all.

Questions (for Alan's sample)

1. Compare Alan's discourse coherence when he describes a school routine and a baseball game. Look at topic maintenance, informativeness, referencing, and fluency (describe and judge whether each feature is appropriate, variable, or inappropriate). Which is more coherent? Which is less coherent? Why are there differences between the topics?

School routine:

Topic maintenance:

Informativeness:

Referencing:

Fluency:

Baseball routine:

Topic maintenance:

Informativeness:

Referencing:

Fluency:

2. What do the differences suggest for intervention with Alan?

Questions (for Robin's sample)

1. Compare each sample for the following. Judge whether each is appropriate, variable, or inappropriate:

Topic maintenance:

    Conversation:

    Narrative:

Informativeness (Is enough information presented; is it presented clearly?)

    Conversation:

    Narrative:

Referencing [Look at personal pronouns (e.g., *she, he, it*)].

    Conversation:

    Narrative:

Fluency:

    Conversation:

Narrative:

2. What are appropriate intervention goals for Robin?

3. What do the differences in discourse coherence among the four genres elicited from Alan and Robin (description of a routine, description of a game, conversation, and personal narratives) suggest about assessment and procedures for intervention?

17

Test/Task Performance versus Discourse Analysis

Clinicians generally evaluate test behavior and conversational discourse when assessing a child or adult. Test data and conversation represent two different types of behavior. Test items are structured and decontextualized (i.e., the absence of setting or uniform topic) while discourse is less structured and has a context.

Each assessment procedure has advantages and disadvantages. Tests are usually easy to administer and score; they provide normative data that are useful if a child is compared with peers of the same chronological age. They help determine if there is a discrepancy between a child's score and those of his peers (Paul, 2001). However, test scores are limited. They do not establish baseline performance, identify goals for intervention, or measure progress in discourse (Paul, 2001). Test behavior may not be representative of the child's communicative abilities (Dever & Gardner, 1970). A child may perform better on a test than in discourse because it is more structured. On the other hand, a child may perform poorly on a test because there is no natural context. Also, poor test-taking skills, hyperactivity, and distractibility diminish test performance. Many tests evaluate isolated abilities that do not reflect natural conversational skills.

Analyses of discourse samples are informative because functional communication abilities are assessed. A clinician determines how well a child actually communicates. However, discourse analyses are limited because of the absence of normative data and standardized procedures. They are also time-consuming to transcribe and analyze.

Both types of evaluation measures are needed, in addition to other measures, for a complete assessment. Criterion-referenced measures are designed to assess specific behaviors that were not elicited on a test or in a language sample. While normative data do not exist for these measures, they enable clinicians to obtain specific information. In the exercise in this section, one criterion-referenced task was used to evaluate specific syntactic structures. Other nonstandardized measures can assess metalinguistic and other abilities. Congruence between different assessment measures and the clinical judgments of a child's abilities does not always occur (Aram, Morris, & Hall, 1993). Objective and subjective information needs to be considered; language assessment is both an art and a science (Allen, Bliss, & Timmons, 1981).

Assessment Applications

1. Clinicians need a variety of assessment measures, including tests, discourse analyses, and criterion-referenced tasks.

2. Variations in performance may occur on different tasks. Clinicians need to consider the difficulty of each task when comparing behavior among different measures.

3. Clinicians should use their clinical judgment in addition to standardized and nonstandardized assessment measures to evaluate language abilities. For example, children may earn scores that are appropriate for their age and be considered to be an inadequate communicator. The reverse may also be true (e.g., failing test scores and appropriate communication skills).

Intervention Applications

1. Goals for intervention should be identified on the basis of multiple assessment measures.

2. Functional communication, rather than test behaviors, should be the focus of intervention. Tests cannot be used to determine goals for discourse (Paul, 2001).

3. Intervention tasks need to be contextualized (e.g., in natural settings and functional discourse topics) in contrast to decontextualized tasks that are found on most standardized tests.

Introduction to the Sample

Aaron is enrolled in a self-contained classroom for children with specific language impairment. His scores on intelligence tests fall within average intelligence as measured by nonverbal testing.

Aaron
9 years, 2 months

Test/Task Data

The Test of Language Development-Intermediate (Hamill & Newcomer, 1982):

    Sentence combining: standard score*, 3; percentile**, 2

        Task: Combine two sentences into one (e.g., *She picked an apple. She ate an apple.*)

        Characteristics: standard score, 6; percentile, 9

        Task: *All birds are blue.* True or false?

        Word ordering: standard score, 1; percentile <1

        Task: Put these words in a sentence: *big am I*

        Generals: standard score, 5; percentile, 5

        Task: How are these words alike, Venus, Mars, and Pluto?

        Grammatic comprehension: standard score, 8; percentile, 25

        Task: Is this sentence "correct?" *Me play ball.*

Spoken language quotient***: 64 (all five scores are totaled)

Listening quotient: 85 (Characteristics + Grammatical comprehension)

Speaking quotient: 59 (Sentence Combining + Word Order + Generals)

Semantic quotient: 76 (Characteristics + Generals)

Syntactic quotient: 66 (Sentence Combining + Word order + Grammatical comprehension)

Test of Auditory Comprehension of Language—Revised (Carrow-Woolfolk, 1985)

Word classes & relations:	12th percentile
Grammatical morphemes:	28th percentile
Elaborated sentences:	23rd percentile
Total score:	18th percentile

Peabody Picture Vocabulary Test—Revised (Dunn & Dunn, 1981): 42nd percentile

Test of Word Finding (German, 1989): Lower than the 1st percentile

Aaron's responses were often characterized by long latencies, substitutions, and insertions, which expressed word-retrieval deficit, such as *I know but . . . like, whatcha call it?* and *I forgot.*

---

*A standard score is a transformation of a raw score (Hamill & Newcomer, 1982). It indicates in standard deviation units the degree to which a child's score deviates from the average score of a group of children. For each subtest at each age level, the mean score is 10 and the standard deviation is 3. In the test manual for the second edition (Hamill & Newcomer, 1982) the following interpretation guidelines are presented for the standard scores on the subtests: 0–2 = poor; 3–6, below average; 7–13, average.

**A percentile is a score on a scale of 100. It indicates the percentage of children at or below each score. A rank at the 10th percentile would indicate that only 10 percent of the sampled population scored below the child's score. The higher the percentiles, the better the performance.

***The following guidelines are presented in the test manual of the second edition (Hamill & Newcomer, 1982) for all quotients: 50–69 = poor; 70–84 = below average; 85–115, average.

Criterion-Referenced Task: On a nonstandardized language task designed to study syntactic ability, Aaron omitted noun and verb inflections, copulas, and auxiliaries. He substituted present tense for irregular verb tense (e.g., *come* for *came*).

Discourse Sample

Adult: Tell me about your cats.

1. A couple of days ago, when we moved into this one house, there's bunch of cats and caught one outside and 2. there was the kitten 3. and I had it for two years and 4. it had babies and um 5. it didn't have a black cat 6. but they had a gray and had a gray cat. 7. We called that Bright Eyes 8. be' [cause] uh that the first cat what opened it eyes 9. and this other one was so sick he wouldn't either walk. 10. He hadta be alone and everything. 11. My other cat, he just wouldn't let other . . . ,12. maybe couple of times, 13. but he wouldn't . . . 14. and um but my my . . . 15. When uh they had them, he came right back to them after. 16. We put, we put my big cat in a house 17. name Tiger 18. and um we put, we . . . 19. When we came right home, he was laying on, um my mom bedroom floor. 20. Uh We don't like laying on bedroom floor. 21. Know why? 22. It so much blood laying on the floor 23. and she wanted to put uh like uh I don't know, like a towel, just then a rag away or something and um 24. she, and um, she had them right in there. 25. um My mom won't let uh girls see them 26. but . . . I, she let me 27. because uh I'm uh one what catch him. 28. Like for three years I been trying to catch that cat, kitten, 29. and um my mom just wouldn't just wouldn't let uh girls go in. 30. Mom, I don't know what, uh . . . 31. sometimes she scratches and stuff. 32. That what I don't know.

Questions

1. Aaron's test data suggest reduced syntactic ability (see summary of test and task performance). Compare his performance on the tests and task to his spontaneous language abilities with respect to:

   a. Sentence combining (conjoined sentences with *and, but, because*).

Test/task performance summary:

Discourse:

   b. Use of copulas:

Test/task performance summary:

Discourse:

   c. Use of the past, plural possessive and third person inflections:

Test/task performance summary:

Discourse:

   d. Word Retrieval:

Test/task performance summary:

Discourse (look at the presence or absence of dysfluencies):

2. Does Aaron show a lack of knowledge of syntax in your opinion? Why?

3. The tests and task that were used do not analyze discourse coherence. Analyze Aaron's discourse coherence with respect to:

   a. Topic maintenance:

    b. Informativeness:

    c. Referencing and lexical usage:

    d. Fluency:

4. Is there agreement among the different assessment measures? Support your answer.

5. (a) Based solely on the test/task data, what would be your goals for intervention with Aaron? (b) Based on the discourse sample data, what would be your goals? (c) Based on both sources of information, what would be your goals for intervention?

18

Assessment of Conversational Discourse

The purpose of this chapter is to provide a discourse analysis that is designed to describe the dimensions of language and communicative functioning, rather than to focus on one feature, as has been undertaken in previous chapters. This overall assessment provides a more complete understanding of a child's verbal abilities. In this chapter, *discourse* will be used as a general term that will encompass all aspects of verbal production (except for the sound system). The general term, discourse, is used instead of "language behavior" because discourse is considered to be the organizing foundation of language function (Owens, 1999). *Pragmatics* is the component that organizes and frames the other aspects of language.

The model that will be used in this chapter is the classic framework described by Bloom and Lahey (1978). It is used because it is practical, concise, and comprehensive. The interrelated dimensions of use, form, and content are employed to describe communicative functioning. These categories are useful for describing language impairments to nonprofessionals, such as teachers and parents, because they are easily understood (Nelson, 1998).

Use refers to pragmatics, the communicative intent or conversational acts that may be expressed, and also discourse. Form refers to structure of sentences, morphology, and the sound system. Content refers to the meaning inherent in utterances. These components frequently interact with one another. More than one component is often disrupted in language pathology.

The following issues should be considered regarding discourse analyses:

1. The guidelines presented in this chapter are suggestions for one approach to a conversational analysis. There are other approaches that are more complete or are comprised of different analyses (see Lund & Duchan, 1993; Nelson, 1998; Paul, 2001; Retherford, 1993).

2. A major purpose of an overall assessment is to describe a speaker's strengths and weaknesses. In this chapter, only one source of information is used, the results of a conversational discourse analysis. Data from case history questionnaires and interviews, psychometric results, standardized assessment measures, different discourse genre analyses, and behavioral observations are needed to complete an assessment protocol.

3. A critical component of an assessment protocol is the evaluation of auditory functioning, which is not addressed in this chapter. Standardized tests and criterion-referenced measures are used to evaluate this important aspect of communicative functioning.

4. Within the three categories of use, form, and content, I have presented suggestions for specific analyses. All of these questions do not need to be answered. Clinicians will need to determine the extent of their assessment and the types of questions that are relevant. Analyses may vary with different children. For example at the presentence level (MLU between 1.0 and 2.50) conversational acts (e.g., assertives and responsives) and semantic relations are typically assessed (Carrow-Woolfolk & Lynch, 1982). At higher levels of MLU, when sentences emerge, discourse, use and content abilities are evaluated (Carrow-Woolfolk & Lynch, 1982).

5. The purpose of this analysis is to describe a child's discourse function. The etiology of each impairment cannot be determined on the basis of only a discourse analysis. More information is needed in order to identify a cause of the language impairment, such as test data, psychometric scores, and evaluations from other professionals.

6. The analysis in this section is different from the ones that have been done in previous chapters in that summary statements regarding different areas are made. The identification of specific utterances by their numbers is not performed because the analysis is more general—appropriate for a report. You will see that the utterances are not numbered in the samples that are provided in this chapter. The statements in the answers are descriptive and represent summaries of behavior, rather than analyses of specific utterances. In my opinion, an overall assessment, in particular one that will be presented to other professionals, should be concise and easy to read. The detailed previous analyses that you have done have laid the groundwork for the more general approach that is used in this chapter.

Assessment Applications

1. Assessment should be comprehensive and cover use, form, and content or pragmatics, syntax, morphology, semantics, and phonology.

2. Assessment is not concerned only with errors that a speaker makes. Clinicians need to focus on a child's strengths as well as the communicative strategies that may be used (e.g., circumlocutions for word-retrieval deficits; overgeneralization of rules that signal their knowledge, *mans* and *comed*).

3. Errors need to be considered within a communicative context. For example, the clinician needs to ask, "Does the error impair the communication of a speaker's meaning (e.g., deletion of actions or objects) or is the error primarily of form (e.g., *me* for *I*)? Does the speaker make his or her needs known?"

Intervention Applications

1. Intervention targets should initially consist of forms that are emerging, those that are not produced inappropriately all of the time (Fey, 1986).

2. Goals should be based on their functionality (e.g., use in a variety of natural contexts), ability to be modified upon stimulation, and frequency of use.

3. Focused stimulation is an effective intervention procedure. The clinician models specific grammatical structures in natural contexts (Cleave & Fey, 1997; Fey, 1986). The goal is to highlight targeted forms for the child. Examples are presented in Part Five of this book.

Introduction to the Samples

Shewann and John are 4-year-old African American children. Billy and Yvette are European North American children. Additional information is not presented so that the reader can make independent decisions about each child's communicative functioning.

Shewann

4 years, 1 month

Clinician: See what's in there [a box with objects].

Shewann: What these?

C: Let's look.

S: What these do? Eat it [sees a picture of cheese].

C: It's cheese.

S: Look, the block [points to a set of blocks].

C: Look what else I found [carton of milk].

S: Milk.

C: What do we do with the milk?

S: Pour it on.

C: Pour it on what? Your head?

S: [shakes his head to indicate no] Pour it.

C: [shows a toy horse] What does the horse do? [makes the horse walk]

S: Horsie go.

C: Does he walk?

S: No, run.

C: See what else I have.

S: Baby [baby doll] . . . down . . . Roll [makes the baby roll over].

C: Oops. What happened [doll's leg came off]?

S: Leg.

C: He broke his leg. What should I do?

S: Let me [reaches for the doll so he can attach the leg].

C: What are you going to do to him?

S: Put his leg on. See?

C: Good job. Oh, what happened? [doll's head came off]

S: Head off [Shewann puts the boy in the fire engine].

C: The boy's gonna drive the fire engine

S: No, he not.

C: Yes, he's gonna drive it to the fire. Then what does he have to do?

S: Climb here [points to the fire engine].

C: Now what?

S: Get horse out. Climb.

C: Climb?

S: No, throw water on it.

C: Where's the water?

S: Right here [points to the hose on the fire engine]. Pick it up.

C: With what? Can I carry the water in my hands?

S: Yeah.

C: What do I need?

S: More. Allgone fire.

C: [moves fire engine to the station house] Now let's go back to the station house.

S: Yeah, right here [points to station house]. Head off [head fell off the doll again].

C: Head off again?

S: Yeah, hair off.

C: Hair off too?

S: Yeah, broke leg [the doll's leg came off]. See, leg [touches the other leg, which is attached]. Look, head on [puts on the doll's head].

John

6 years, 10 months

John: Know Marty on *Back of Future*?

Clinician: Yes, did you see the movie?

J: No, me see it on tape.

C: Tell me about *Back to the Future*

J: Me watch that movie before with my real parents. Marty go way up in the sky with Doc.

C: Was it *Back to the Future I*?

J: No, Two. One on tape.

C: Do you know that *Back to the Future III* is out now?

J: Yes, no.

C: Are you gonna see it?

J: Me see that with my real parents before.

C: Can I help you with these? [play children and school bus]

J: Where they going?

C: To school. Do they have to drive in a car to go to school?

J: No, they have the bus. The bus take 'em down school.

C: Which one [of the people toys] is the teacher?

J: The teacher a girl?

C: She's got dark hair just like me. Which one is Mrs. Jones? [his teacher]

J: Mrs Jones a girl?

C: Mrs Jones is a woman.

J: Me only, me only find one girl.

C: Well, how about this one?

J: That one, that one gonna be a teacher.

C: Yes?

J: Them gonna be a teacher, Mrs. Jones.

C: OK.

J: Him [one of the other toy people] gonna be a kid.

C: Yeah, but that's mine.

J: Yeah, see him bigger.

C: Is that a boy?

J: Yep, that me right there.

C: That one looks like the father.

J: Um that not a father. He have a hat. Maybe that gonna be me.

C: OK, That's gonna be John.

J: Me fighting the bad kid.

C: I don't think the bus driver is gonna let you on the bus if you're fighting.

J: Tell me uh name of that kid right there.

C: How about Ben?

J: No, me don't want that.

C: How about calling him, Doc?

J: Doc, Doc a man.

C: Who's this?

J: Me. John wanna play with them [picks up two of the toy people].

C: Where are they going?

J: Them going on a trip.

C: Are they going to Seaworld?

J: Yes, on a boat. Them [points to some of the toy people] going. Them [points to other toy people] going with them.

C: Who else is going? Is this guy going too?

J: Yeah, no.

C: He should go. Let's see. Put him here in this car.

J: Why I'm a bad kid?

C: You're not a bad kid. Do you want to name them?

J: Doc a man.

C: Who's Doc?

J: Doc ride in the *Back of Future* car.

Billy

10 years

Clinician: How old are you?

Billy: Ten.

C: You're ten?

B: I been going to her past a year.

C: Have you always been going to this school?

B: Yep. We're never gonna move out it, of our house.

C: How come?

B: 'Cuz um . . . there's lots of memories in at our house. I fall asleep at ten.

C: How do you know that?

B: Easy. I count uh, I look . . . I got a clock in my room but it says ten o'clock. You can tell they took out the clock in here [no clock in the therapy room].

C: Yep, they sure did.

B: 'Cept they left the clock in there [points to another room] 'cuz we using that room because she wants, the one that owns this room here, she wants hers in there.

C: Her what?

B: Um where they hang up their coats. They hang up their coats in there [points to another room]. They had a table in here. They took it out. They left it crooked.

C: How come?

B: They're too lazy. One fell asleep. The other one stayed awake.

C: Who?

B: The janitors. One fell asleep and pushed down one end. The other one's awake, holding up the other end.

C: How do you know that happened?

B: Easy, I was watching 'em. I was spying.

B: Anymore questions?

C: What?

B: Anymore questions?

C: Why, are you tired of talking?

B: Talking about one thing.

C: What do you want to talk about?

B: Anything you want.

C: Like what?

B: Speech.

C: What do you do in speech?

B: She teaches us. Sometimes um we play games.

C: What kind of games?

B: um Like choo choo.

C: Can you teach me how to play choo choo?

B: Take three chairs [he puts three chairs in a row]. Have a . . . whoever gets it right, they move up. Whoever gets it wrong, has to move to the back.

C: What does Ms. Smith [the speech-language pathologist] do?

B: She asks us sentences or . . .

C: Does she say a sentence and you have to say it back?

B: She says it wrong. We hafta say it right. That's how we hafta say it.

C: What else do you do?

B: Ummmm, oh, like Cat. Gotta see if it's a boat, choo choo, or an animal.

C: What's it called?

B: Cat, if it's a boat, a stuffed animal, or animal.

C: I don't get it.

B: You hafta choose A, B, or C.

C: Oh, if she says, "Cat?"

B: Cat, you hafta say it. um If, words, that I just said and you hafta choose "C."

Yvette

15 years

Clinician: What did you do in Idaho?

Yvette: I went I went to [different state] and um my aunt um had these snakes and I watched it eat up these mice and then um she let it out loose by accidentally and I and I I slept on the floor 'cause so that's the highest spot and I like snakes and well kinda little bit scary and um she, it climbed all over me and it went down here and tickled me and I screamed and my aunt rushed in the room and the snake bit her in the eye and it bit me in the leg, right here [points] and I had to be going to the hospital and then we went to my friend's house and my aunt's other one, that lives by her . . . and they, she wait. The next door neighbor had a dog that had babies I didn't know that dogs bite when they have babies and I go and the boy threw the purse by the dog and I went and got it and the dog came, shout out um like, "you won't take my little babies," and um I went over there and he bit me in the same spot and I almost died but I didn't and because the um I . . . and and in 15 more minutes I would have been dead and then um after that I went back to my aunt's house and the snakes were gone. I didn't want to go asleep and they caught one of them. It didn't bite me yet. It bit my aunt in the eye and then two time and she she had to go to the hospital have surgery done on her eye and she said that um she's gonna get rid of them but she never did and she she was gonna give me one but I go, "no way" 'cause I have a little sister coming 'cause now I have another. My ma's having another baby . . . June, in June.

C: Did you get bitten by the snake and the dog both on the same days?

Y: No, not on the same day, different weeks.

C: Does that dog live next door to you at home?

Y: Yeah.

C: Or where your aunt lives in [name of a state]?

Y: In [her home state]. We came back and we went there for for um a while and then and they had to take me to the doctor. I have a scar in my leg. I'll show you. It's not very far up. It's just right down, right there [points] and it hurt and I was crying and blood came shooting out and my little cousin . . . we . . . it was in the spring or in summer. Well, I don't know but um [sigh] after I was going back to my house um there's these dogs that were loose and and and I . . . 'cause a few days later, like . . . yesterday or something, um we slept at a community building for scouts and my friend, Heidi, she told these boys to come and pound on the wall.

[Some background information is needed for this sample. This conversational sample was elicited in the same manner as the previous ones. Yvette elaborated on her answers more than the other children. Most of the information that Yvette provided is true. However, she was bitten by a dog and not by a snake. One of her aunts had eye surgery but not as the result of a snakebite.]

Questions

Follow the format presented below to describe the communicative functioning of the children. All of the questions do not need to be answered; use your own judgment regarding those that are most relevant for a particular child. Summarize the child's functioning in each section. Do not refer to specific utterances. The goal of this section is to enable you to describe the overall abilities of each child.

Assessment of Conversational Discourse

1. Use

   A. Is the child an active conversationalist? Does the child express a variety of assertives and responsives? Is the child actively engaged in the conversation? Sometimes children do not ask questions in a discourse sample. However, a speaker can be judged to be an active communicator because the child answers questions readily, elaborates responses, or responds positively to the clinician in the discourse. This analysis is most appropriate for children at the presentence level.

   B. Is the child's discourse coherent (i.e., characterized by appropriate topic maintenance, informativeness, and referencing)? This analysis is most appropriate for children using sequences of sentences.

   C. Is the child's production generally fluent? (Some dysfluencies should be expected since they occur in everyone's verbal production.) Are there excessive abandoned utterances, internal corrections, repetitions, pauses, and fillers?

2. Form

   A. Syntax
      (1) Does the child have an appropriate utterance length? (The answer does not always need to be made on the basis of quantifying mean length of utterance.) Does the child use a variety of grammatical categories including verb-related forms—such as, auxiliaries, copulas, modals, and adverbs—and noun-related forms—such as nouns, adjectives, prepositions, pronouns, possessives, and demonstratives?
      (2) Does the child use a variety of grammatical structures (e.g., simple and complex sentences)?

   B. Morphology
      (1) Does the child use word endings? (e.g., the inflections of plural, past, possessive, and third-person singular).
      (2) Does the child use grammatical irregular verbs and noun forms?

   C. Phonology (not the focus of this book)

3. Content

   A. Vocabulary use
      (1) Does the child use a diversity of words? (The answer in this book will be subjective rather than a quantitative analysis.)
      (2) Does the child use words appropriately (e.g., are there examples of errors of word usage or too general words that do not have specific meanings)?

   B. Does the child exhibit knowledge of agents and objects by expressing some of the following concepts: attribution, quantification, spatial and location, mental states, possession, and mental states? Note that the expression of some of these concepts will be determined by the topics of conversation. Absence of a concept does not mean lack of understanding of its meaning. Semantic relations will generally be identified at the presentence level, and diversity of relations will be identified when a child is using sentences.

C. Does the child exhibit knowledge of actions and events by expressing the following concepts: temporal relations, causality, and manner?

4. What are the child's strengths and weaknesses?

5. What are your conclusions regarding the nature of the child's language development, based on the analysis of the sample (remember that test scores, case history information, and observations should also be used)?

6. What are your recommendations for the child (e.g., enrollment in intervention, implementation of a parental program, reassessment in six months)? If intervention is recommended, what goals are appropriate for the child?

Assessment of Conversational Discourse

Child's name: **Shewann**   **Age: 4 years, 1 month**

USE

FORM

CONTENT

STRENGTHS AND WEAKNESSES

CONCLUSIONS

RECOMMENDATIONS

Assessment of Conversational Discourse

Child's name: **John**   **Age: 6 years, 10 months**

USE

FORM

CONTENT

STRENGTHS AND WEAKNESSES

CONCLUSIONS

RECOMMENDATIONS

Assessment of Conversational Discourse

Child's name: **Billy**   **Age: 10 years**

USE

FORM

CONTENT

STRENGTHS AND WEAKNESSES

CONCLUSIONS

RECOMMENDATIONS

Assessment of Conversational Discourse

Child's name: **Yvette**   **Age: 15 years**

USE

FORM

CONTENT

STRENGTHS AND WEAKNESSES

CONCLUSIONS

RECOMMENDATIONS

Part Five

Intervention

The purpose of this section is to describe an interactive approach to language intervention that is based on functional communication (Bliss, 1993; Owens, 1999). In this approach, discourse is the foundation for intervention. The rationale of the interactive approach is that many children with language disorders do not spontaneously use their linguistic knowledge to communicate (Johnston, 1985). Use of behaviors that have been mastered in a structured clinical setting has not been achieved spontaneously. Children with language disorders do not often generalize behaviors, because they are unable to apply rules flexibly in different contexts (Kamhi, 1998). Intervention activities are needed to promote generalization learning and transference from the clinical setting to functional communication. To achieve generalization, intervention should incorporate conversational acts and functional contexts (Kamhi, 1998).

The following guidelines reflect the interactive intervention approach. They should be considered after a child has gained a basic knowledge of a linguistic structure or pragmatic behavior.

Guideline 1): Develop natural contexts. Realistic communicative situations need to be utilized in intervention programs to achieve meaningful interactions. Structured exercises may not always promote generalization of new behaviors to functional communication (Owens, 1999). Learning in context facilitates language acquisition (Nelson, 1998; Owens, 1999; Paul, 2001).

Implementation: Incorporate natural contexts, such as mealtime, shopping, eating at a restaurant, and taking a trip.

Guideline 2): Use meaningful communication. Meaningful communication consists of conveying new information to a listener. Individuals are motivated to convey novel and interesting information (Hudson & Shapiro, 1991). When a clinician and a child are looking at the same picture while the child describes it, meaningful information is not conveyed, since both participants see the same referent.

Implementation: Enable a child to describe new information to the clinician.

Guideline 3): Use discourse-based feedback. The highest form of reinforcement is communication (Mahoney, 1975). Intervention activities should be developed in which communication of information is recognized and rewarded. Extrinsic reinforcement, such as "good job," is not discourse-based.

Implementation: When the child gives an appropriate utterance, comment or elaborate on the content of the child's utterance. With inappropriate responses, use contingent queries or repeat the inappropriate utterance to enable a child to revise what was said. For example:

Child: *Me go home*
Clinician: <u>Who</u> *went home?*
Child: *I go home.*

To determine whether an activity is interactive, the clinician should answer the following questions:

1. Is there a natural context?
2. Is meaningful communication used?
3. Was discourse-based feedback used?

Consider the following excerpt from an intervention session.

Clinician: [puts a ball on a table] Where is the ball?
Child: On table.
Clinician: [puts a pencil in a box] Where is the pencil?
Child: On box.
Clinician: It is IN the box. Where is the pencil?
Child: In box.
Clinician: Good talking, it is IN the box. [clinician puts a block under a book] Where is the block?
Child: There [points to the block].
Clinician: No, tell me where it is.
Child: [points and says] Book.
Clinician: It is UNDER the book. Where is the block?
Child: Under.
Clinician: Say the whole thing.
Child: Under book.
Clinician: Good talking.

The following questions should be answered to determine whether this activity is interactive:

1. Is there a natural context?
   No, different objects are used; there is no unifying topic for discussion.
2. Is meaningful communication used?
   No, both the clinician and the child see where the objects are placed; no new information is exchanged.
3. Was discourse-based feedback used?
   No, the clinician does not elaborate or comment on the child's appropriate utterances and does not use contingent queries with inappropriate responses.

This task could have been made interactive if there had been a unifying topic or theme, such as a meal.

The child could have been requested to place objects in and on plates, bowls, cups, and a table. Meaningful communication would also occur if the child directed the clinician to place the objects in different locations. The clinician would have elaborated on the child's appropriate responses and asked clarifying questions when the child answered inappropriately.

Initially, focused simulation activities are useful to enable a child to understand concepts attached to various aspects of language behavior (Cleave & Fey, 1997; Fey, 1986). A clinician models a syntactical structure or discourse function by providing numerous examples. The child is not requested to say anything. For example, an adult can frequently use adjectives in many natural contexts. The goal is to provide maximal stimulation for these forms. Later, activities are designed to elicit production of adjectives. Focused stimulation procedures facilitate the production of simple and complex language forms (Cleave & Fey, 1997; Fey, 1986). In Part Five we will focus on elicited production. Further examples of focused stimulation are found in Fey (1986) and Cleave and Fey (1997). In chapters 19 and 20 two aspects of form and content are highlighted. Verb and noun phrase expansion is elicited with adjectives and modals. These two grammatical categories were selected because they represent a combination of form and content. Both represent syntactical categories; they also embody meaning or content. The modals can and cannot express the concepts of ability and inability adjectives reflect attribution that can express a diversity of meanings. These two grammatical categories are vulnerable in language pathology and are frequent targets in intervention (Bliss, 1993).

The remaining two chapters highlight the "use" or pragmatic category of communication. The focus is on two of the four categories described by Grice (1975). In Chapter 21, the category of relation is addressed with topic maintenance. In Chapter 22 the category of quantity is highlighted with respect to informativeness. These two discourse dimensions were selected because they also are frequently impaired in childhood language disorders. They are critical for coherent discourse and academic success.

19
Intervention: Modals

Modals are necessary to produce grammatical negatives and questions. They also represent a diversity of meanings, such as ability and permission for *can*; intentionality for *will*; obligation for *should*; and possibility for *may* and *could*. They should be elicited after a child produces agent + action + object structures (Bliss, 1993).

In this exercise we will focus on ability with *can* and inability with *cannot*. Some intervention guidelines with respect to modals are (Bliss, 1993):

1. Place modals initially at the end and later at the beginning of utterances to increase their saliency.

2. Make modals critical to a situation by incorporating their meaning into a natural context. *Can* and *can't* should be elicited with respect to their meanings of ability and inability by having the child become aware of actions an individual can or cannot perform. The same concept is relevant for intentionality with *will* (e.g., child discovers activities that will or will not be performed).

3. Pair modals with their opposites to highlight their meaning.

Sample Exercise

Initially, focused simulation activities are useful to enable a child to understand the concepts attached to modals (Fey, 1986). For the words *can* and *can't*, natural contexts are developed in which the clinician demonstrates the ability or inability to perform a variety of activities. For example, a clinician could try to open a tightly closed jar and could say, *I can't open it*. Then the adult could get a kitchen tool and loosen the jar and say, *Now I can*. After the child has been familiarized with the targeted modals and their concepts, production activities can be implemented. An example of an activity that is designed to elicit the modals *can* and *can't* with ability and inability is presented below.

Goal: Increase the production of modals that represent ability and inability

Context: Snack.

Procedures and instructions: Provide relevant items for a snack, such as juice (water), cookie, tightly or loosely closed jar of peanut butter, tightly closed or loosely closed jar of jelly, cracker, and glass.

The clinician presents the context by saying, *I'm hungry. I hope you are. Let's have a snack.* The clinician places an empty glass in front of the child and says *Can you drink the juice (or water)?*

With an inappropriate response (e.g., if the child only says *no* or does not respond), the clinician says, *No you can't. There's no juice. You can't drink. You can say, "No, I can't drink."* Then the clinician pours some juice (or water) in the glass and asks, *Now, can you drink?* If the child does not respond or only says *yes*, the clinician can say, *Yes you can. There is some juice (water). You can drink.*

You can say, "Yes, I can." This procedure allows the clinician to model the desired responses *I can* and *I can't*.

With an appropriate response, the clinician expands and comments on the child's utterance (e.g., *there is no water, you can't drink; you need some water* or *you have water, you can drink it*).

This procedure should be repeated with additional items with sample questions, *Can you eat? Can you open it?* (tightly versus loosely closed jar of peanut butter or jelly).

As a modification, the objects can be placed behind a barrier so that only the child can see whether there is juice (or water) in the glass. Then the clinician can ask the same questions. In this context the child will provide new information because the clinician supposedly does not know whether the child can or cannot perform the task.

After the child has mastered the structures, *Yes, I can* and *No, I can't*, a verb can be added (e.g., *Yes, I can eat, No, I can't eat*). Finally, the objects can be interspersed to elicit a variety of structures (e.g., *No, I can't eat, Yes, I can open it*).

Question

Develop a similar exercise with appropriate items and utterances for modals *can* and *can't*.

Context:

Procedure and instructions:

20
Intervention: Adjectives

Attribution is important because it enhances the following aspects of language development (Bliss, 1993; Owens, 1999):

(1) Semantics. The use of adjectives reflects and expands concept development; children can acquire new concepts and then use adjectives to represent their meanings.

(2) Syntax. The use of adjectives serves to elaborate sentence structure by expanding the noun phrase.

(3) Pragmatics. Adjectives increase informativeness; they enable a speaker to specify referents in simple sentences and relative clauses.

In intervention, meaningful contexts are developed in which an adjective is critical for conveying specific information. Focused stimulation activities would be appropriate prior to the elicitation of adjectives. For example, an adult can show a child two objects that are different with respect to one feature (e.g., red ball and blue ball). The adult comments on the differences in the objects by highlighting the contrasting feature. Additional objects are presented to the child and their contrasting features are modeled by the clinician. Later, the child can be asked to comment on the differences between objects.

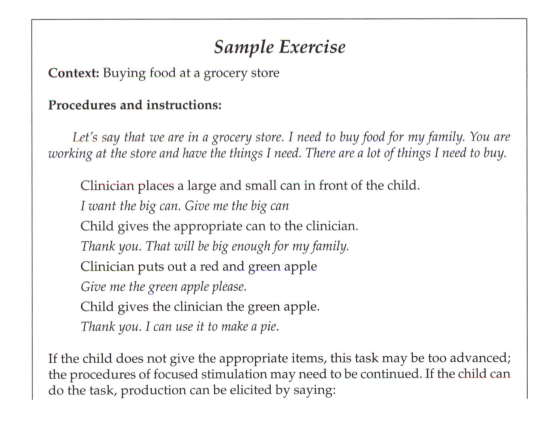

Sample Exercise

Context: Buying food at a grocery store

Procedures and instructions:

Let's say that we are in a grocery store. I need to buy food for my family. You are working at the store and have the things I need. There are a lot of things I need to buy.

Clinician places a large and small can in front of the child.

I want the big can. Give me the big can

Child gives the appropriate can to the clinician.

Thank you. That will be big enough for my family.

Clinician puts out a red and green apple

Give me the green apple please.

Child gives the clinician the green apple.

Thank you. I can use it to make a pie.

If the child does not give the appropriate items, this task may be too advanced; the procedures of focused stimulation may need to be continued. If the child can do the task, production can be elicited by saying:

Now pretend you are going to do the shopping. Here are two potatoes. It's your turn to ask me for one of them. You can say, "Give me the ___."

Sample items:

large and small can
red and green apples
red and brown potatoes
yellow and green bananas
round and square cookies

large and small cookies
chocolate and white milk
round and square crackers

Question

Develop a similar exercise with appropriate items and utterances for a different context.

Context:

Procedure and instructions:

21
Intervention: Topic Maintenance

Listening, auditory comprehension, and topic maintenance are closely associated. Deficits in topic maintenance reduce discourse coherence because a speaker cannot be easily understood if a topic is not sustained. Off-topic utterances indicate that a child does not understand a previous utterance or topic or is inattentive (Owens, 1999).

Topic maintenance should be elicited in a natural context and by providing a child with a motivation to maintain a topic. Verbal redirection is a discourse-based procedure that will assist a child in attaining this goal. (Lucas, 1980) When a child provides an appropriate response, the clinician repeats the question, answers it, and then asks the question again. In this way, the appropriate response is modeled. Activities should be structured in which topic maintenance is inherent in a context (Brinton & Fujiki, 1989). A child can be instructed to talk about a topic for a specific purpose, such as ordering something from a catalogue or solving a problem (Brinton & Fujiki, 1989).

Sample Exercise

Context: Selecting an appropriate gift

Procedures and instructions:

The clinician will say:
> *Pretend that it is Christmas time. You need to buy a lot of gifts.*
> > *What gift would you buy your friend, [name of child], and your mother?*
> > *Why would you buy your friend that gift?*
> > *Why would you buy your mother that gift?*
> > *What is the difference between the gifts?*
> > *Why would your friend like the gift?*
> > *Why would you mother like her gift?*

With an appropriate response (e.g., *I'd buy Jamie a CD and my mom a book*), the clinician will comment on the response by agreeing with the child or expanding the thought (e.g., *I bet Jamie would like a CD* or *What one would you get her?* and *Your mom likes to read; she would like a book*).

With an inappropriate response (e.g., *I want my own phone*), the clinician can first ask a contingent query (e.g., *What would you buy Jamie? What would you buy your mother?*) If the child continues to go off topic, the clinician can ask the original question, give a possible answer or some choices the child can select, and then ask the question again (e.g, *What would you buy Jamie and your mother? I might buy Jamie a CD and your mother a book. What would you buy Jamie and your mother?*)

Here are additional questions that can be asked:

Now you need to buy your cousin and your aunt a gift.
What gift would you buy your cousin and your aunt?
Why would you buy your cousin that gift?
Why would you buy your aunt that gift?
What is the difference between the gifts?
Why would your cousin like the gift?
Why would your aunt like her gift?

Sample items:

The procedure can be repeated with the following contrasts of purchasing gifts:

Your mother and your father

Your cousin and your aunt

Your teacher and your friend

Question

Develop a context and procedures designed to elicit topic maintenance.

Context:

Procedures and instructions:

22

Intervention: Informativeness

Speakers need to provide their listeners with sufficient information so they can understand them. Informativeness refers to the amount of information that a speaker provides to a listener; it is critical in informal situations and also in academic contexts. Children with language disorders do not always provide enough information for a listener to understand what they are saying (Miranda, McCabe, & Bliss, 1998). Their messages are unelaborated, and critical information is omitted. Focus on this discourse dimension is needed both in clinical contexts and in classroom settings. Collaborating with teachers is critical to improve informativeness.

In this section, informativeness will be elicited in two communicative acts during conversational discourse. Responsive communicative acts will be highlighted to enable children to provide sufficient information to the listener when questions are posed. Informativeness will also be elicited in assertive communicative acts with the production of directions. The child will need to provide sufficient information when giving directions to someone.

Informativeness is elicited with discourse-based feedback. When a child provides a response or direction that has sufficient information, the clinician elaborates, comments, or expands upon the child's utterance. When the child leaves out information the clinician can either ask a clarifying question (contingent query) to enable the child to provide additional information or direct the child to provide more information (e.g., by saying, *Tell me more*).

Responsive Conversational Acts

In this section, answers to questions will be elicited. The responsibility of the speaker is to provide enough information for the listener to understand a message. To increase informative responses to questions, clinicians provide a topic in discourse and ask the child relevant questions.

Examples of tasks that are designed to elicit informative responses:

1. Topic of conversation (context): zoo
   Clinician: Have you ever been to a zoo? With an affirmative reply, the clinician will ask the child the following questions:

   What animals are in the zoo?

   Where do they live?

   Who takes care of them?

   Why do we have zoos?

   How do we take care of the animals?

   Why do we go to zoos?

2. Topic of context (context): story
   Clinician: It was Janey's birthday. She was going to have a party. She wanted a kitten for her birthday.

   Who would be invited to the party?

   What games would be played?

   How is one of the games (that the child mentions) to be played?

   What would there be to eat at the party?

   Why does Janey want a kitten?

   Where would the party take place?

These two activities involve meaningful communication because information is exchanged. The child needs to create novel answers to the questions.

Assertive Conversational Acts

One type of an assertive conversational act is giving directions. Procedural discourse involves a description of the steps necessary to carry out an activity.

There are easy and more difficult forms of procedural discourse. Easier forms of procedural discourse involve fewer steps and more concrete (e.g., visible) actions. More difficult types of procedural discourse are characterized by additional and more abstract (e.g., nonvisible) steps.

Some examples of directions with their critical steps (you may have identified additional components of each task) are:

Easier directions:

I'm hungry. I like peanut butter and jelly sandwiches. My mother always makes them. I want to make one. Can you tell me how to make a peanut butter and jelly sandwich?

Steps: (1) Get out two pieces of bread; (2) put peanut butter on them (or one slice); (3) put jelly on both or one slices; and (4) put slices of bread on each other. Optional step: Cut the sandwich.

More difficult directions:

Let's plan a surprise birthday party for your friend. Tell me how to plan the party.

Steps: (1) Decide who will be invited, the date, time, and location of the party; (2) make appropriate arrangements; (3) determine how to keep the party a secret; (4) plan how to get the person to the party; (5) determine what to eat; (6) identify the entertainment; and (7) agree on an appropriate gift; and (8) determine other arrangements.

Questions

1. Responsive conversational acts
   Describe a topic of conversation and relevant questions that would elicit informativeness.

2. Assertive conversational acts
   Develop two activities that are designed to elicit informativeness with directions. List the required information for these activities.

   a. Describe an easy task:

   b. Describe a more difficult task:

Part Six

Answers for Selected Chapters in Text

Chapters 2, 4, 6, 8, 10, 12, 14, 16, 18, 20, 22

Chapter 2

1. Identify examples of assertive and conversational acts from Cameron's sample.

Assertive Conversational Acts

Requests for information: 20, 21
Requests for action: 13, 15, 16*, 17*, 22*, 23, 24, 26*
Comments: 3, 6, 7, 8*, 10*, 11, 14, 18, 19, 25, 28, 29, 30
Statements: 1, 5, 9
Total number of assertives: 23

Responsive Conversational Acts

Answers: 1, 2, 4, 12, 27
Action responses: none
Statement responses: None
Total number of responses: 6

Other

Other: 0
Total number of other: 0

*Some ambiguous utterances and my rationale for codings.

8: I consider this utterance to be a comment because Cameron is describing the bubbles that he blew; he is not requesting more bubbles.

10: could also be considered as a response to the clinician's question.

16, 17, 22, 26: Are these responses to requests for information, requests for actions or even comments? I have interpreted them as requests for action. In #16, the adult interprets Cameron's utterance as a request; when she says *There*, she assisted the child in blowing up the balloon. In #17, I interpreted the child's utterance to mean [Yes, make it go] *more up*, which would suggest a request for action. Without this interpretation, the utterance could be interpreted as a spontaneous comment/description of the location of the balloon or as a response to a statement [again, with *yes* implied]. In #22, the utterance could be: (a) response to the clinician's question, with an implied *yes*, (b) a request for action, or (c) "other" because it could be an echolalic utterance (however, Cameron does not show other tendencies of echolalia). In #26, similar issues are raised. Note that the clinician's previous ut-

*This utterance is ambiguous; the utterance may suggest, *Can it stay up here?* This interpretation would be coded as a missing modal.

terances elicit a request for action as she said *Do you want?* Before each of these utterances.

2. Based on your analysis, what type of communicator is Cameron? Support your answer.

Cameron is an active conversationalist. He produces a variety of assertive and responsive conversational acts. In my opinion he engaged freely and actively with the clinician.

3. Does Cameron need intervention to increase his repertoire of conversational acts? Support your answer.

I would not work on increasing his conversational acts at this time, although he does not show many responses to statements. He needs work on expanding his utterance length and other aspects of language structure (see next section).

4. List two intervention goals for the following conversational profiles.

Passive conversationalist:
  a. Increase requests for information and action.
  b. Elicit comments and statements.
Inactive communicator:
  a. Elicit assertive and responsive conversational acts.
  b. If there are deficits in auditory comprehension, or speech intelligibility that contribute to the reduced interaction of the child, focus on these impairments.
Verbal noncommunicator:
  a. Increase topic maintenance.
  b. Focus on listening, auditory comprehension, and attention that may contribute to this profile. Behavioral management may be necessary.

Chapter 4

1. Verb phrase expansion is especially vulnerable in language pathology. Identify the utterances in which there is presence or absence of the copula, auxiliary, modal, and auxiliary *do/does*.

copula verb present: 4, 22
copula verb absent: 6, 10, 11, 12, 13, 15, 17, 18, 19, 20, 21, 23, 24, 25, 26
auxiliary verb present: none
auxiliary verb absent: 2, 5, 29
modal auxiliary present: 9
modals present: none
auxiliary *do/does* present: none
Auxiliary *do/does* absent: 3*, 28

2. Why might Craig's usage of *where's* and *that's* be learned forms (memorized utterances)?

Because the copula appears only with these forms

(4, 22). It is absent in the other obligatory contexts (see above). Craig might be in the process of learning the copula and has begun to use it with *where* and *that*. Additional sampling is needed to determine whether these are truly learned forms or represent emergent mastery.

3. Identify utterances characterized by either the presence or absence of articles, adjectives and possessives and demonstratives before the noun.

Presence article + noun*: none*
Absence of article: 4, 10, 11,12, 20
Presence of adjective before noun: none
Presence of possessive before noun: 7, 18, 19
Presence of demonstrative before noun: 12, 24

4. Perceptual saliency may influence the language production of children with language disorders. In this sample, compare Craig's use of articles versus demonstratives. How might perceptual saliency affect his performance?

Demonstratives are more salient (e.g., pronounced, noticeable) than articles. Salient forms are generally used more often by children with language impairment than forms that are reduced in saliency (Leonard, 1998). However, there are other influences than perceptual saliency. For example, there is a difference in performance between the plural and the third-person singular *s*, the former is used more than the latter in early stages of language development and in language pathology (Rice & Oetting, 1993). The influence of the verb also influences language production; verbs are more difficult than nouns for children with language disorders (Watkins, 1994).

5. What would be your goals for intervention?

I would elicit an increased number of modals and adjectives. Copulas, auxiliaries, and articles are reduced in perceptual saliency and meaning. I would reserve these forms until other salient aspects of language structure have been acquired. I would not focus initially on the ungrammatical pronouns (e.g., *him/he, him/his, her/she*) until Craig has increased his verb and noun phrase development.

Chapter 6

1. Describe Michael's ability to use the following dimensions of discourse coherence, as described in this section.

Topic maintenance:

Cartoon (utterances 1–8):

Michael is on topic in this sequence.
Pumpkin pie (9–12):
He is on topic in these utterances although he give tangential information (e.g., 10, *something nasty*, 11 and 12, *tasted like black*) . He does not respond appropriately to questions that involve time (9, 10).
Halloween (13–22):
Michael is on topic in utterances 13–15. He is off topic in utterances 16–22; his utterances appear to reflect associations.
Batman movie (23–41):
Michael gives on-topic responses.

Informativeness (what information is present and what information is missing?):

Cartoon (1–8):
Michael includes information about the actions of the witch, owl, and pumpkin.
Michael omits information about the setting (where did the action take place?) and internal states (why did the witch stick her thumb in her hand? Why did the owls say *Pumpkin pie*? Why did the pumpkin run?).
Halloween (13–22):
Michael describes the initial events of trick or treating. He omits the result of saying *Trick or treat*.

Referencing:

Personal referencing (utterances 2, 6, 15, 17, 19):
Appropriate: *She* (2, witch); *they* (6, owls), *we* (15, me and my brother).
Inappropriate: *Sherri* (17, the listener does not know who Sherri is), *they* (19, the listener does not know the referent for this pronoun).
Fluency: (identify the dysfluencies) :
Abandoned utterances: 6, 20, 27, 31, 37, 38
Fillers: *um/er*: 17, 20, 24, 29, 34, 40 (Note: We all use fillers to some degree; this usage probably does not reduce Michael's discourse coherence.)
from: 10, 29, 30, 37, 38
Like: 1, 11, 12, 29, 30

Note: *From* is used appropriately in 1 (*something nasty from this witch*) and 10 (the second use, *something nasty be coming from pumpkin seeds*). *Like* is used as a comparison in 3 (*she go like this*), maybe in 11 and 12 (*like black*, what do you think?), 35 (*it's like a bat*) and 36 (*it's like a light*). I have not seen the movie. I may be less able to understand what Michael is trying to convey than someone else who has seen the movie. Do you agree?

Summarize Michael's discourse coherence:

Strengths: topic maintenance and referencing (although he has some difficulties in this area).

Weaknesses: Informativeness and fluency.

Overall discourse coherence: Variable. The main ideas of what Michael conveys can be understood; the listener will not be able to obtain specific information.

2. How well will Michael do in school? Support your answer.

Michael will do poorly because he is limited in providing specific information. His answers to questions in class will be too general. His dysfluencies will also decrease his discourse coherence.

3. What intervention goals would you identify for Michael? Why did you select them?

I would initially target informativeness and referencing. Michael needs to provide more information for the listener in order to be coherent. Although his referencing is sometimes appropriate, I would focus on this aspect to enable him to be more consistent with referencing. I would not focus on fluency, it may improve with increased informativeness. If not, then fluency can be approached by encouraging Michael to plan his utterances before he speaks.

4. It is critical to integrate Michael's intervention with his classroom activities and discourse. How would you integrate them?

a. The speech-language pathologist should work as a consultant and collaborator with Michael's teacher. The clinician should encourage Michael's teacher to do the following:

(1) Ask contingent queries when a child is not providing a coherent utterance.

(2) Model answers for a child.

(3) Simplify a task for a child who has difficulty responding; instead of asking general questions or those that require explanations, the teacher can ask for specific information or use questions that require limited responses.

b. The speech-language pathologist can visit the classroom and observe how well a client is performing. The clinician can model suitable questions for a teacher to ask.

Chapter 8

1. Rudy's deficits are primarily in the area of discourse rather than syntax. Describe his perfor-

mance with respect to the following dimensions of discourse:

Topic Maintenance: Appropriate

Rudi stays on the topic throughout this discourse. His answers are on the same topic as the clinician's questions.

Informativeness: Variable

Some of Rudi's utterances are informative although they may be incomplete (utterances 1, 2, 5, 8, 9, 12, 13, 30, 31, 32, 33) . His gestures help us understand some of what he is saying. While it is not always possible to easily understand what Rudi is trying to communicate, the gist or essence of his utterances can generally be understood. However, some of his utterances are not coherent (e.g., 19, 20, 23, 24, 26). You might have considered Rudi's informativeness to be inappropriate; this judgment would also be acceptable. It is difficult to make a definitive decision for this discourse dimension.

Referencing: Inappropriate

Appropriate use: the demonstratives, *here, there, this,* and *that* (utterances 2, 4, 6, 35, and 36) are clarified with Rudi's pointing gestures. *It* (utterance 15) refers to his desk.

Inappropriate use: *before that* (utterance 22); *stuff happens* (utterance 22); 23, *who moved the desk?*; *they* (utterance 28); *you* (utterance 29, Rudi means a student or some barrier).

References not stated but understood by the context: *it* refers to Rudi's desk in many utterances (7, 11, 14, 28).

Fluency: Inappropriate

Abandoned utterances: 19, 24, 26

Internal correction: 7 (some people have said that this utterance is an abandoned utterance, it could be)

Pauses: 7, 16, 19, 24, 26

Fillers: *Um*, 23; *like*, 2, 3, 4, 5, 11, 15, 17 (first usage), 23 (two examples), 27, 29. Note there are three appropriate uses of *like* (utterances 12, 17, 18).

2. What intervention goals would be appropriate for Rudy?

Increase informativeness.

Elicit appropriate referencing.

Enable Rudy to concisely describe an event.

3. What communication behaviors will be difficult for Rudy in his classroom (e.g., following complex directions)?

Answering questions concisely and coherently.

Presenting coherent oral reports.

Participating in group discussions.

4. Social impairments are also evident in adolescent language learning disorders. What impairments in social interaction might an adolescent with language learning disorders exhibit?

Unpopularity.

Could be overly aggressive because of frustration at not being popular or not being understood.

Isolation

Recipient of teasing and taunting.

Lack of knowledge of slang words that serve as social links to peers.

Chapter 10

Immediate Echolalia

1. Identify the 18 echolalic utterances in Evan's sample.

1. 1: Made a ball
2. 4: Snow ball
3. 6: Another car
4. 8: It's blue
5. 9: I make a snake
6. 11: Bracelet
7. 14: More stuff
8. 15: Make a house
9. 16: This color house
10. 17: It red
11. 18: Color roof
12. 19: White
13. 20: Square house
14. 25: Dry out
15. 26: Go in
16. 30: A bird
17. 32: Some lunch
18. 35: White soup

Note that Evan repeats mostly the last portions of previous utterances. He may be using the echo as a means to understand the clinician's utterances.

2. Provide support for the claim that Evan has limitations in understanding the word *color* and the concepts it represents.

Evan repeats a number of utterances in which the word *color* is used (e.g., 16,18) or specific colors are mentioned (8, 17, 19, 35). Note, also, that he repeats utterances with quantifiers—*another* (6), *more* (14), and *some* (32). This pattern suggests that Evan does not understand the concepts in utterances that he repeats.

3. Does Evan echo more statements than questions? What is the significance of this finding regarding Evan's communicative competence?

Yes, the only questions that Evan echoes are 15, 16, 18, 19, 26, and 32. He answers questions [2, 5, 7 (although it is not appropriate), 22, 27, 28, 31, 33, 34]. The significance of this finding regarding Evan's communicative competence is that he can distinguish between questions and statements. Questions are an easier form for generating a response than statements. Evan has the ability to distinguish between these two forms.

4. What intervention goals would you have for Evan?
   a. Improve comprehension and spontaneous production of semantic relations (see chapter 3) and simple sentences.
   b. Increase comprehension and spontaneous production of colors and quantifiers.

Delayed Echolalia

1. Identify the different examples (e.g., themes or topics) of delayed echolalia (chunks of memorized forms).
   Ghost with the most: 1, 2, 3, 24
   Nintendo Entertainment System: 4, 9, 10, 20
   Of the Lost Nintendo: 21
   World of Nintendo: 22, 23

2. What would be your intervention goals for Kevin?
   a. Improve auditory comprehension, establish a hierarchy, and proceed from simple *wh-* questions to more complex questions followed by statements.
   b. Improve topic maintenance.

3. Do you think that Evan or Kevin is more communicatively impaired? Why?

Kevin is more communicatively impaired, in my opinion. Evan can communicate, although he echoes and uses simple utterances. Kevin's syntactic and vocabulary development is more advanced than Evan's. However his discourse coherence is more limited.

4. In your opinion, does the language development evident in autism reflect a delay or a qualitatively different pattern of development? Why?

The language development reflects a qualitatively different pattern even though children with typical language development show some echolalia. However, in echolalia there is an extreme frequency of occurrence of this typical tendency. The persistent and pervasive echolalia in autism is not found in typical language development. It represents a gestalt processing style, in which structures are not analyzed but are repeated as a whole (Prizant, 1982). Children with typical language development rapidly move from this style to a more analytical processing mode. Children with autism maintain the gestalt style (Prizant, 1982).

5. It is critical for the professional to provide information regarding echolalia to the significant others of a child with autism. What information do you need to provide about echolalia to parents and teachers?
   a. Echolalia is not a willful act of defiance or misbehavior.
   b. Echolalia is a function, in part, of auditory comprehension deficits.

c. Echolalia has communicative and cognitive functions.

d. Individuals should respond to the communicative intent of the echolalic response.

e. Echolalia should not be punished or ignored.

f. Individuals should simplify and shorten utterances that are echoed.

Chapter 12

1. The contradictions in some of Leslie's utterances appear to reflect a difficulty with the self-monitoring aspect of impaired executive function. If Leslie monitored her utterances, she would be able to detect and correct contradictions in her production. Where do contradictions occur in Leslie's utterances?

Utterances 2 versus 3: the contradiction is with *do* versus *did* housework.

Utterances 22 versus 26: the contradiction is whether her mother is mad or not mad at her.

Utterances 9, 10 11, 12: the contradiction is whether the grandmother is going to leave or stay.

2. Leslie's concreteness is evident in her reduced semantic development. For example, she does not completely understand and produce causality concepts expressed with *because*. What utterances are characterized by impaired comprehension and/or production of causality (note in 22 that her use of causality is appropriate)?

26, 27, 29 (the answer is incomplete; it may be appropriate), 39, 41, 42

3. Leslie's impulsivity and lack of attention span are evident in her abrupt changes of topic. She cannot disinhibit her impulses, so she talks about whatever comes to mind without making transitions. Usually the new topics are related by associations to the former topics. Where do you notice abrupt changes of topics?

4, 21, 23, 30, 35, 37, 39

4. What would be your intervention goals (consider both executive function and communicative effectiveness) for Leslie?

Executive function goals:

Improve planning and organizing discourse and self-monitoring behaviors.

Decreasing disinhibition.

Communication goals:

Increase discourse coherence and reduce topic shifting.

Increase the knowledge of the concept of causality.

5. Describe a task that would incorporate the goals of improving both executive function and communication. Show how both aspects would be involved in an intervention task.

The task is to prepare a surprise party for Leslie's grandmother. We need to begin by making preparations; this task would elicit planning and organizing behaviors required for effective executive function. The communication aspect would require Leslie to invite people, order food, and explain why we are having the party. In these tasks, Leslie would be encouraged to monitor and regulate her discourse.

Another task that involves both executive function and communication is narration, in which events, movies, or books are described. A speaker needs to organize a message that will be communicated and to regulate discourse so that the message will be coherent.

Chapter 14

Jose

1. Where are there the following SiE features in Jose's discourse?

Present tense for irregular past-tense verbs

Fight/fought: 1, 3   *fights/fought*: 2 (also overgeneralization of third-person singular form)

Tell/told: 10   *get/got*: 4

Bleed/bled: 7 (there are two types of misusage in this utterance: the word *bleed* cannot be used to convey cause and there is a tense error)

Absence of inflections:

Cry/cried: 6

Know/knew: 12 (this is somewhat ambiguous; the tense may be appropriate)

Substitutions of prepositions:

At/to: 3

On/to: 9

2. Jose also uses English versions of these and other non-SiE features. Show where.

Use of irregular verbs: *said*: 11, 12; *went*: 8; *came*, 9, *hit*: 5

Use of the copula and auxiliary:

Copula *was*: 11

Auxiliary *was*: 1, 5, 10

Use of inflections:

Past *ed* (*called*), 5

Use of subject pronouns: *I*: 1, 2, 7, 10, 11, 12; *he*: 3, 8; *we*: 4; *she*: 10

3. Are there utterances that do not appear to represent SiE? They may reflect incomplete mastery of English, use of a child's unique rule system, or a language impairment. If so, identify these utterances.

2: *I fights with him* (overgeneralization of third person singular)

7: *I bleed him* Jose means to say ("make him bleed")

10: absence of object pronoun (*her,* . . . *she tell* [ ] *that I was fighting* . . .) this utterance may reflect colloquial (informal) use).

These utterances reflect Jose's ability to form his own rules and usage. Not all L-2 usage is based on L-1 usage.

Chapter 14

Juan

1. Where are there SiE features in Juan's discourse?

Present tense substituted for past tense:

Go/went: 3, 11, 20, 25, 30

Sting/stung: 13 (child may not have learned this infrequent word)

Take/took: 21

Get/got: 29

See/saw: 9, 19 (incomplete utterance), 20

Absence of inflections:

Past *ed: finish* (5; this utterance is difficult to interpret), *close* (6), *stay* (18), *jump* (22)

Third-person singular *s: like,* 26

Absence of subject pronouns: 13, 25

Absence of copulas and auxiliaries (including the perfective):

Them crawling: 10; *We fishin',* 15; *We calling,* 22; *Them not,* 25; *Them already* [had] *gone* (perfective usage or absent copula, *were gone*)

Substitutions of prepositions:

On/at, 18 *on/in,* 9, 10 (My students do not always agree that these are substitutions.)

2. Juan also uses English versions of these and other non-SiE features. Show where.

Use of subject pronouns (Although they may be ungrammatical, the subject is presented.):

Me: 2, 4, 7 etc.

Them: 10, 11, 12, 14, 24, 25, 28

It: 8, 9

We: 15, 18, 20, 21, 22

He: 23 (incomplete)

Use of inflections:

Plural *s:* 17, 18, 20; Third-person singular: 28

Use of irregular verbs:

got, 2, 14, *hit,* 12

Use of copulas:

8, 9

3. Are there utterances that do not appear to represent SiE? They may reflect incomplete mastery of English, use of a child's unique rule system, or a language impairment. If so, identify these utterances.

Pronoun substitution

Subject for object: *Me/I:* 2, 4, 7, 9, 27, 29, 30
    Them/They: 10, 11, 12, 14, 24, 25, 28
Repetitions: 5, 6, 8, 14, 20 (they may have been used to emphasize a point).
Excessive pauses: 1, 5, 10, 11, 13, 18, 19, 20, 22, 23, 26 (Although they may be signs of second language learning, Juan pauses to find the appropriate English word.)

4. What would be the reasons for enrolling Juan in an intervention program and what are the reasons against enrolling him?

The issue is whether Juan's language behavior reflects limited English proficiency or whether there is a language impairment. He has failed two tests of language proficiency, in his native language and in English. However, current tests are very limited in their value (Restrepo, 1998). It would be better to base the decision to enroll Juan on the quality of the language samples in both Spanish and English, and to look at the number of grammatical errors per T-Unit as well as the length of T-Unit in Spanish (Restrepo, 1998). Since he is language impaired in both languages, as reported by the family, teacher, and a bilingual speech-language pathologist, I think he should be enrolled in therapy to increase his language effectiveness in both languages. A bilingual speech-language pathologist should work with Juan.

Chapter 14

David

1. Show where David is dysfluent.
    Abandoned utterances: 1, 2, 6, 7, 8, 9, 10, 11, 12, 13
    Repetitions: 8, 14
    Excessive pauses: 1, 2, 5, 6, 7, 8, etc.
    Internal corrections: 2 (this utterance could also be an abandoned utterance).

Fillers: 1, 2, 5, 6, 8, 12
2. Where does he show inappropriate referencing?
4: Who is *somebody*?
5: We do not know who Danielle is.
9: Who is *the man*?
14: Is the girl Danielle?
15: What is the referent for *his*?
3. What utterances cannot be clearly understood?
8, 15

Chapter 16

Alan
1. Compare Alan's discourse coherence when he describes a school routine and a baseball game. Look at topic maintenance, informativeness, referencing, and fluency (describe and judge whether each feature is appropriate, variable, or inappropriate). Which is more coherent? Which is less coherent? Why are there differences between the topics?
School routine:
Topic maintenance: Appropriate
All of his utterances focused on the school routine.
Informativeness: Variable
Alan gives only sketchy information; he does not provide details about school. He gives the "gist" of the information without elaboration; he does not mention his classes, for example. He may not have known that more details would have made his message easier to understand.
Referencing: Appropriate
Many references are understood by the context of Alan's discourse: *we* (2, 3, 4, 5, understood as students), *here* (4, understood as the residential school), *they* (6, understood as adults).
One example of inappropriate usage: *we* (6, omission)
Fluency: Variable
Dysfluencies: repetition (2, 5), revision (5, *have* for *watch* or the utterance could have been intended to be *have* [*to*] *watch*, that would not represent a revision) and pause (7).
Baseball routine:
Topic maintenance: Appropriate
All of his utterances focused on the baseball game.
Informativeness: Inappropriate
It is difficult for the listener to follow the procedures of the game. Details are missing, such as the goal of the game and the team membership.

Referencing: Inappropriate.
Inappropriate usage: we do not know the referents for: *the guy* (9), *in the middle* (9, of what?), *it* (10, a ball?), *they* (10, the hitter?), *the other guy in the middle* (12), *him* (13), *that way* (13, what does this mean?), *he* (13), *circle* (13, where is it?), and *he* (twice in 14).
Appropriate usage: *the guy* (11, the hitter), *he* (12, the hitter)
Fluency: Variable
Abandoned utterances (9,12), revision (10, it is still not clear) and pause (12) at the end of the utterance
Alan's description of his school routine is more coherent than the description of the baseball game. The routine consists of listing of activities, which is a relatively simple task. The description of the baseball game involves planning and organizing discourse. Alan is limited in his ability to produce a complex coherent message that involves planning and sequencing.
2. What do the differences suggest for intervention with Alan?
Alan should describe short simple events, such as familiar routines and actions. Discourse complexity can be increased gradually by adding length and more difficult tasks, such as describing other sports activities and personal experiences (e.g., vacations).

Robin

1. Compare each sample for the following features. Judge whether each is appropriate, variable, or inappropriate.
Topic maintenance:
Conversation: Appropriate
Robin stayed on the topic of the trip to Colorado.
Narrative: Appropriate
Robin described one incident. At the end of the narrative he talked about doors, which are related to the topic of the hospital.
Informativeness (Is enough information presented; is it presented clearly?)
Conversation: Appropriate
Enough information was presented for the listener to understand the facts pertaining to Robin's trip to Colorado; the only exception is with utterance 1, where he talks about throwing rocks in the sea. The listener needs more information to understand Robin's meaning in this utterance.
Narrative: Inappropriate
There are contradictions: *broke leg* versus *dog bite* (16, 17) and *hit the dog* versus *pour water on it* (29, 30) and missing information: what is the significance of

the doors opening (34, 35, 37)? What happened to his sister?

Referencing [Look at personal pronouns (e.g., *she, he, it*)].

　　Conversation: Appropriate

　　Their (4, people in Colorado), *her* (6, sister), *we're* (8, 9, 13, 14, 15, Robin, father and sister), *he's* (11, boss)

　　Narrative: Variable

　　(Who had the dog bite, the mother or the sister? I assume it is the sister because the question asks about the sister, however it could be the mother.) The referencing changes depending on whom you think was bitten. My students have never reached agreement on the identity of the person.

　　What we know for sure:

　　Appropriate: *she* (16, sister), *her* (17, 18, sister), *she* (21, 28, 29, mother) and *it* (21, dog)

　　Possible interpretations: *she* (22, dog) and *that* (22, bites)

　　Inappropriate: we do not know the identity of the subject of Robin's narrative: *her* (23, mother or sister) and *she* (32, 34 and 36, mother or sister)

Fluency

　　Conversation: Variable

　　There are some pauses (1, 4, 5, 7, 9, 10, 11) and two repetitions (4, 10). Most of Robin's conversation is fluent.

　　Narrative: Inappropriate

Pauses (19, 25, 31, 33), repetitions (19, 21, 25, 32), fillers (17, 19, 24, 25), and abandoned utterances (25, 33)

2. What are appropriate intervention goals for Robin? Increase discourse coherence. Use a hierarchy from simple to more complex discourse. Have Robin describe simple routine activities and procedures, proceed to short (and then extended) descriptions of past events (personal narratives). Increase referencing and informativeness.

3. What do the differences in discourse coherence among the four genres elicited from Alan and Robin (description of a routine, description of a game, conversation, and personal narratives) suggest about assessment and procedures for intervention?

The clinician needs a variety of discourse genres to evaluate communicative competence. Conversation is generally not demanding enough for all children. Children need to be challenged by more difficult discourse genres in order to identify their impairments.

Chapter 18

Child's name: Shewann　　**Age:** 4 years, 1 month
USE

　　Shewann was an active conversationalist. He requested actions and information. He spontaneously described events and answered questions.

FORM

　　Shewann's utterance length was short for his age. He used most frequently nouns, verbs, verb particles, prepositions, and pronouns in simple sentences. Modals, adjectives, and prepositions were absent. Auxiliaries, copulas, and word endings were absent, either as a result of African American English or a language pathology.

CONTENT

　　Shewann used a limited number of semantic relations. He produced most frequently action + object structures. There were no agent + action + object forms.

STRENGTHS AND WEAKNESSES

　　Shewann's strengths were his ability to actively engage in conversation and to make himself understood. He was limited in his utterance length, semantic relations, and variety of grammatical categories and sentence structures.

CONCLUSIONS

　　Shewann is impaired in language development for his age, based on this discourse sample.

RECOMMENDATIONS

　　Shewann should be enrolled in individual and group intervention programs. The goals should be to: (1) increase production of agents, (2) elicit agent + action + object structures, and (3) stimulate modals, adjectives, and prepositions after simple sentences have been acquired.

Child's name: John　　**Age:** 6 years, 10 months
USE

　　John was an active conversationalist. He made spontaneous requests for information and comments. He responded readily to the clinician's questions. His utterances were generally coherent. He did not always answer questions appropriately; he may have impairment in auditory comprehension.

FORM

　　John used simple sentences with a variety of grammatical categories, including nouns, verbs, adverbs, prepositions, pronouns, and articles. He did not use complex sentences, modals, past-tense irregular verb forms, and a variety of adjectives. His uses of the pronouns *I, they,* and *she* were ungrammatical. Omission of auxiliaries, most copulas, and some word endings may represent use of African American English or a language pathology.

CONTENT

John used the following concepts: temporal relation of past tense, location, quantification, and possession. Absence of additional concepts (e.g., causality and mental states) may have been the result of the nature of the topics that were discussed. He appears to have limited attribution, the use of adjectives to describe people and objects; however his ability in this area should be studied further.

STRENGTHS AND WEAKNESSES

John's strengths were his abilities to actively engage in a conversation and to use simple sentences. He was limited in the grammatical production of most pronouns and did not use a variety of adjectives and modals. He did not use complex sentences.

CONCLUSIONS

John is language impaired for his age.

RECOMMENDATIONS

John's auditory comprehension and his knowledge of attribution should be assessed. He should be enrolled in a language intervention program with the following goals: (1) elicit modals and grammatical production of pronouns, (2) model complex sentences, and (3) assess his auditory comprehension and his ability to use a variety of adjectives.

Child's name: Billy   **Age:** 10 years

USE

Billy was an active conversationalist, although he asked only one question. He readily answered questions and made spontaneous comments. Billy's discourse was not consistently coherent because he did not always provide sufficient information for the listener to identify the people and actions that he mentioned. His discourse was generally fluent.

FORM

Billy's syntactic skills were adequately developed; he used both simple and complex utterances with a variety of grammatical categories, word endings, and irregular verb forms.

CONTENT

Billy used a variety of words and concepts, including quantification, past tense, possession, causality, location, and attribution.

STRENGTHS AND WEAKNESSES

Billy's strengths were his active conversational style and his syntactic and semantic competence. His discourse coherence was reduced; he did not always completely identify people and actions in his conversation.

CONCLUSIONS

Billy's communicative abilities are impaired for his age because of his reduced discourse coherence.

RECOMMENDATIONS

Billy should be enrolled in an intervention program with the goal of increasing discourse coherence. He needs to be able to provide sufficient information for a listener to fully understand him. The goal of intervention should be to increase the informativeness of his messages by adequately describing individuals and actions.

Child's name: Yvette   **Age:** 15 years

USE

Yvette was an active conversationalist, although she did not ask any questions. She responded readily to the questions posed by the clinician. Several of her answers were very long and rambling and included tangential and associative thoughts. Even though Yvette provided lengthy answers, she did not always give sufficient information for the listener to understand her discourse. She omitted critical information about people, locations, and events. A listener would be able to understand the overall meaning of her discourse; the details would be difficult to grasp. Yvette embellished some of the information that she described. Although her utterances were generally fluent, some repetitions, pauses, and incomplete utterances were evident.

FORM

Yvette used simple and complex sentences with a variety of grammatical categories. She made occasional syntactic errors that were not consistent and did not reflect a lack of knowledge of syntactic forms.

CONTENT

Yvette used a variety of words to express a range of concepts, including past tense, location, manner, attribution, and possession. Her use of causality was variable. Sometimes her use of the word *because* did not reflect the concept of causality; it was sometimes used as a filler, to maintain her discourse.

STRENGTHS AND WEAKNESSES

Yvette's strengths were her active conversational style and her syntactic and semantic competence. She was limited in the ability to produce concise and coherent messages. She did not always provide sufficient information for the listener to understand her discourse.

CONCLUSIONS

Yvette is language impaired because of her reduced discourse coherence.

RECOMMENDATIONS

Yvette should be enrolled in an intervention program that is designed to increase her discourse coherence. The goal should be to produce concise messages in which sufficient information is presented to a listener. Her speech-language pathologist needs to collaborate with her classroom teachers to help her increase her coherence in classroom activities that involve oral communication.

Chapter 20

Develop a similar exercise with appropriate items and utterances with a different context.

Context: Packing for a trip

Procedures and instructions:

The clinician places two items of clothing in front of the child that contrast in at least one feature (see below for examples) and a suitcase. The clinician would say (the wording can be changed to suit the vocabulary level of the child):

Let's pretend you are going on a trip. Here is a suitcase. You need some clothes. I will pack this suitcase for you. You need to give me some clothes.

Clinician places a yellow shirt and red shirt before the child.

Give me the red shirt.

Child packs the appropriate shirt

This is a nice shirt. It will look good on you.

Clinician puts out a big sock and a small sock.

You need something to wear on your feet. Give me the big sock; it will fit you.

Child packs the appropriate sock.

Yes, you will need the big sock. The small sock won't fit you.

Clinician puts out red tie and a blue tie.

Now I have the clothes. You will pack them. You need to ask me for one of them. You can say, "Give me the red tie."

Proceed with different items (e.g., different colors of dresses, slacks, socks, shoes, ties; and different sizes of shirts, hats, jackets, and belts).

Chapter 22

1. Responsive conversational acts

Describe a topic of conversation and relevant questions that would elicit informativeness.

Topic (context): Tim was late for school.

Questions:

Why was he late?

What are other reasons he could have been late?

What will happen to him?

What should he say to his teacher?

Why will he never be late again?

2. Assertive conversational acts.

Develop two activities that are designed to elicit informativeness with directions. List the required information for these activities.

a. Describe an easy task:

Pretend your little cousin needed to mail a letter. She didn't know how to mail one. Tell her how to mail a letter.

Required steps: (1) find paper, (2) write a letter, (3) put paper in envelope, (4) address envelope, (5) write return address, (6) put a stamp on the envelope, and (7) mail the letter.

b. Describe a more difficult task:

Tell me how to play baseball.

Required information: (1) the goal of the game, (2) who plays the game, (3) who are the team members, (4) the responsibilities of each team member, (5) how points are scored, (6) how each team scores points, and (7) the mechanics of the game (e.g., errors, walks, home runs, etc.).

References

Abbeduto, L., & Rosenberg, S. (1992). Linguistic communication in persons with mental retardation. In S.F. Warren & J. Reichle (Eds.), *Causes and effects in communication and language intervention* (pp. 331–360). Baltimore: Paul H. Brookes.

Allen, D.V., Bliss, L.S., & Timmons, J. (1981). Language evaluation: Science or art? *Journal of Speech and Hearing Disorders, 46,* 66–78.

American Psychiatric Association. (1994). *Diagnostic and statistical manual of mental disorders* (4th ed.). Washington, DC.

Anderson, R. (1994). Cultural and linguistic diversity and language impairment in preschool. *Seminars in Speech and Language, 15,* 115–124.

Anderson, R.T. (1996). Assessing the grammar of Spanish speaking children: A comparison of two procedures. *Language, Speech and Hearing Services in Schools, 27,* 303–314.

Aram, D.M., Morris, R., & Hall, N.E. (1993). Clinical and research congruence in identifying children with specific language impairment. *Journal of Speech and Hearing Research, 36,* 580–591.

Aram, D.M., & Nation, J. (1982). *Child language disorders,* St. Louis, MO: Mosby.

Bates, E. (1976). *Language and context: The acquisition of pragmatics.* New York: Academic Press.

Bates, E. (1979). *The emergence of symbols: Cognition and communication in infancy.* New York: Academic Press.

Bedore, L.M., & Leonard, L.B. (1998). Specific language impairment and grammatical morphology: A discriminant function analysis. *Journal of Speech, Language, and Hearing Research, 41,* 1185–1192.

Berman, R., & Slobin, D. (1994). Narrative structure. In R. Berman & D. Slobin (Eds.), *Relating events in narrative: A crosslinguistic developmental study* (pp. 39–84). Hillsdale, NJ: Erlbaum.

Beukelman, D.R., & Yorkston, K.M. (1991). Traumatic brain injury changes the way we live. In D.R. Beukelman & K.M. Yorkston (Eds.), *Communication disorders following traumatic brain injury: Management of cognitive, language and motor impairments* (pp. 1–13). Austin, TX: PRO-ED.

Biddle, K.R., McCabe, A., & Bliss, L.S. (1996). Narrative skills following traumatic brain injury in children and adults. *Journal of Communication Disorders, 29,* 447–469.

Bland-Stewart, L. (2000). Personal Communication.

Bliss, L.S. (1984). The development of listener-adapted communication by educably mentally impaired children. *Journal of Communication Disorders, 17,* 372–384.

Bliss L.S. (1985). A symptom approach to the intervention of childhood language disorders. *Journal of Communication Disorders, 18,* 91–108.

Bliss, L.S. (1988). Modal usage by preschool children. *Journal of Applied Developmental Psychology, 9,* 253–261.

Bliss, L.S. (1989). Selected syntactic usage of language-impaired children. *Journal of Communication Disorders, 22,* 277–289.

Bliss, L.S. (1993). *Pragmatic language intervention. Interactive activities.* Eau Claire, WI: Thinking Publications.

Bliss, L.S., & Allen, D.V. (1981). Black English responses on selected language tests. *Journal of Communication Disorders, 14,* 225–233.

Bliss, L.S., McCabe, A., & Miranda, A.E. (1998). Narrative assessment profile: Discourse analysis for school age children. *Journal of Communication Disorders, 20,* 1–8.

Bloom, L. (1973). *One word at a time: The use of single-word utterances before syntax.* The Hague: Mouton.

Bloom, L., & Lahey, M. (1978). *Language development and language disorders.* New York: John Wiley & Sons.

Bloom, L., Lahey, M., Hood, L., Lifter, K., & Feiss, K. (1980). Complex sentences: Acquisition of syntactic connectors and the semantic relations they encode. *Journal of Child Language, 7,* 235–261.

Bloom, L., Lightbown, P., & Hood, L. (1975). Structure and variation in child language. *Monographs of the Society for Research in Child Development, 40.*

Blosser, J.L., & dePompei, R. (1989). The head-injured student returns to school: Recognizing and treating deficits. *Topics in Language Disorders, 9,* 67–77.

Brinton, B., & Fujiki, M. (1989). *Conversational management with language-impaired children: Pragmatic assessment and intervention.* Rockville, MD: Aspen Publishers.

Brown, R. (1973). *A first language: The early stages.* Cambridge, MA: Harvard University Press.

Brown, R., & Bellugi, U. (1964). Three processes in the child's acquisition of syntax. *Harvard Educational Review, 34,* 133–151.

Bryan, T.H. (1986). A review of studies on learning disabled children's communicative competence. In R. Schiefelbusch (Ed.), *Language Competence* (pp. 227–260). San Diego: College-Hill.

Camarata, S.M., Nelson, K.E., & Camarata, M.N. (1994). Comparison of conversational recasting and imitative procedures for training grammatical structures in children with specific language impairment. *Journal of Speech and Hearing Research, 37,* 1414–1423.

Campbell, L.R. (1993). Maintaining the integrity of children's home communicative variety: Speakers of Black English Vernacular. *American Journal of Speech-Language Pathology, 2,* 11–12.

Campbell, L.R. (1994). Discourse diversity and Black English Vernacular. In D.N. Ripich & N.A. Creaghead (Eds.), *School discourse problems* (pp. 93–131). San Diego: Singular Publishing Group.

Campbell, L.R. (1996). Issues in service delivery to African American children. In A.G. Kamhi, K.E. Pollock, & J.L. Harris (Eds.), *Communication development and disorders in African American children* (pp. 73–93). Baltimore: Paul H. Brookes.

Carr, E., Schriebman, L., & Lovaas, J. (1975). Control of echolalic speech in psychotic children. *Journal of Abnormal Child Psychology, 3,* 331–351.

Carrow-Woolfolk, E. (1985). *Test of Auditory Comprehension of Language—Revised.* Allen, TX: DLM Teaching Resources.

Carrow-Woolfolk, E., & Lynch, J. (1982). *An integrative approach to language disorders in children.* New York: Grune & Stratton.

Chapman, R. (1981). Exploring children's communicative intents. In J. Miller (Ed.), *Assessing language production in children* (pp. 111–136). Baltimore: University Park Press.

Cleave, P.L., & Fey, M.E. (1997). Two approaches to the facilitation of grammar in children with language impairments: Rationale and description. *American Journal of Speech-Language Pathology, 6,* 22–32.

Coggins, T. (1979). Relational meaning encoded in the two-word utterances of Stage 1 Down Syndrome children. *Journal of Speech and Hearing Research, 22,* 166–178.

Coggins, T., Olswang, L., & Guthrie, J. (1987). Assessing communicative intents in young children: Low structured observation or elicitation task? *Journal of Speech and Hearing Disorders, 52,* 44–49.

Conti-Ramsden, C., & Jones, M. (1997). Verb use in specific language impairment. *Journal of Speech, Language, Hearing Research, 40,* 1298–1313.

Conti-Ramsden, G., & Botting, B. (1999). Classification of children with specific language impairment: Longitudinal considerations. *Journal of Speech, Language, and Hearing Research, 42,* 1095–1104.

Craig, E., & Evans, J. (1993). Pragmatics and SLI: Within group variations in discourse behavior. *Journal of Speech and Hearing Research, 36,* 777–789.

Craig, H.K., & Washington, J.A. (1994). The complex syntax skills of poor, urban African-American preschoolers at school entry. *Language, Speech, and Hearing Services in Schools, 25,* 181–190.

Craig, H.K., & Washington, J.A. (1995). African-American English and linguistic complexity in preschool discourse: A second look. *Language, Speech, and Hearing Services in Schools, 26,* 87–93.

Craig, H.K., & Washington, J.A. (2000). An assessment battery for identifying language impairments in African American Children. *Journal of Speech, Language, and Hearing Research, 43,* 366–379.

Craig, H.K., Washington, J.A., & Thompson-Porter, C. (1998). Average C-unit lengths in the discourse of African American children from low-income urban homes. *Journal of Speech, Language, and Hearing Research, 41,* 433–444.

Cromer, R. F. (1991). The development of language and cognition: The cognition hypothesis. In R.F. Cromer (Ed.), *Language and thought in normal and language-handicapped children* (pp. 184–252) Cambridge, MA: Basil Blackwell.

Curtiss, S., Prutting, C.A., & Lowell, E. L. (1979). Pragmatic and semantic development in young children with impaired hearing. *Journal of Speech and Hearing Research, 35,* 373–383.

Curtiss, S., Katz, W., & Tallal, P. (1992). Delay versus deviance in the language acquisition of language-impaired children. *Journal of Speech and Hearing Research, 35,* 373–383.

Damico, J.S. (1985). Clinical discourses analysis: A functional approach to language assessment. In C. Simon (Ed.), *Communication skills and classroom success* (pp. 165–206). San Diego: College-Hill.

Dever, R., & Gardner, W. (1970). Performance of normal and retarded boys on Berko's test of morphology. *Language and Speech, 13,* 162–181.

Dollaghan, C., & Campbell, T. (1992). A procedure for classifying disruptions in spontaneous language samples. *Topics in Language Disorders, 12,* 56–68.

Donahue, M. (1987). Interactions between linguistic and pragmatic development in learning-disabled children: Three views of the state of the union. In S. Rosenberg (Ed.), *Advances in applied psycholinguistics.* Vol. 1 (pp. 126–179). New York: Cambridge University Press.

Dore, J. (1975). Holophrases, speech acts and language universals. *Journal of Child Language, 2,* 21–40.

Dunn, L., & Dunn, L. (1981). *Peabody Picture Vocabulary Test—Revised (PPVT-R).* Circle Pines, MN: American Guidance Service.

Ehrens, B.J. (1994). New directions for meeting the academic needs of adolescents with language learning disabilities. In G.P. Wallach and K.G. Butler (Eds.), *Language learning disabilities in school–age children and adolescents* (pp. 393–417). New York: Merrill.

Ewing-Cobbs, L., Fletcher, J.M., & Levin, H.S. (1985). Traumatic brain injury. In M. Ylvisaker (Ed.), *Head injury rehabilitation: Children and adolescents* (pp. 71–89). Austin, TX: PRO-ED.

Fay, W.H. (1967). Mitigated echolalia of children. *Journal of Speech and Hearing Research, 10,* 305–310.

Fay, W.H. (1975). Occurrence of children's echoic responses according to interlocutory question types. *Journal of Speech and Hearing Research, 18,* 336–354.

Fay, W.H., & Butler, B.V. (1968). Echolalia, IQ, and the developmental dichotomy of speech and language systems. *Journal of Speech and Hearing Research, 11,* 365–371.

Fay, W.H., & Schuler, A.L. (1980). *Emerging language in autistic children.* Baltimore: University Park Press.

Fey, M. (1986). *Language intervention with young children.* San Diego: College-Hill.

Fey, M., & Leonard, L. (1983). Pragmatic skills of children with specific language impairment. In T. Gallagher and C. Prutting (Eds.), *Pragmatic assessment and intervention issues in language* (pp. 65–82). San Diego: College-Hill Press.

Fey, M., & Leonard, L.B. (1984). Partner age as a variable in the conversational performance of specifically language-impaired children. *Journal of speech and Hearing Research, 27,* 413–423.

Fey, M., Leonard, L.B., & Wilcox, K. (1981). Speech-style modifications of language-impaired children. *Journal of Speech and Hearing Disorders, 46,* 91–97.

Freedman, P.P., & Carpenter, R.L. (1976). Semantic relations used by normal and language-impaired children at Stage 1. *Journal of Speech and Hearing Research, 19,* 784–795.

Gerber, A. (1993). *Language-related learning disabilities.* Baltimore: Paul H. Brookes.

German, D.J. (1987). Spontaneous language profiles of children with word-finding problems. *Language, Speech, and Hearing Services in Schools, 18,* 217–230.

German, D.J. (1989). *The Test of Word Finding—Revised.* Austin, TX: DLM Teaching Resources.

German, D.J. (1992). Word-finding intervention for children and adolescents. *Topics in Language Disorders, 13,* 33–50.

German, D.J., & Simon, E. (1991). Analysis of children's word-finding skills in discourse. *Journal of Speech and Hearing Research, 34,* 309–316.

Goffman, L., & Leonard, J. (2000). Growth of language skills in preschool children with specific language impairment: Implications for assessment and intervention. *American Journal of Speech-Language Pathology, 9,* 151–161.

Grela, B.G., & Leonard, L.B. (2000). The influence of argument-structure complexity on the use of auxiliary verbs by children with SLI. *Journal of Speech, Language, and Hearing Research, 43,* 1115–1125.

Grice, H.P. (1975). Logic and conversation. In P. Cole & J.L. Morgan (Eds.), *Syntax and Semantics 3: Speech acts* (pp. 41–58). New York: Academic Press.

Grossjean, F. (1982). *Life with two languages: An introduction to bilingualism.* Cambridge, MA: Harvard University Press.

Grossman, H. (1983). *Classification in mental retardation.* Washington, DC: American Association on Mental Deficiency.

Gutiérrez-Clellen, V.F. (1996). Language diversity: Implications for assessment. In K.N. Cole, P.S. Dale, & D.J. Thal (Eds.), *Assessment of communication and language* (pp. 29–56). Baltimore: Paul H. Brookes.

Gutiérrez-Clellen, V.F. (1999). Language choice in intervention by bilingual children. *American Journal of Speech-Language Pathology, 8,* 291–302.

Gutiérrez-Clellen, V.F., Restrepo, M.A., Bedore, L., Peña, E.,

& Anderson, R. (2000). Language sample analysis in Spanish–speaking children: Methodological considerations. *Language, Speech, and Hearing Services in Schools, 33,* 88–98.

Hadley, P.A. (1998a). Early verb-related vulnerability among children with specific language impairment. *Journal of Speech, Language, Hearing Research, 41,* 1384–1397.

Hadley, P.A. (1988b). Language sampling protocols for eliciting text-level discourse. *Language, Speech, and Hearing Services in Schools, 29,* 132–147.

Hadley, P.A., & Rice, M. (1996). Emergent uses of BE and DO: Evidence from children with specific language impairment. *Language Acquisition, 5,* 209–243.

Halliday, M.A.K., & Hassan, R. (1976). *Cohesion in English.* London: Longman Group.

Hamill, D., & Newcomer, P. (1982). *The Test of Language Development-Intermediate* (2nd ed.). Austin TX: PRO-ED.

Hansson, K., Nettelbladt, U., & Nilholm, C. (2000) Contextual influence on the language production of children with speech and language impairments. *International Journal of Language and Communication Disorders, 35,* 31–47.

Hemphill, L. (1989). Topic development, syntax, and social class. *Discourse Processes, 12,* 267–286.

Hemphill, L., & Siperstein, G. (1990). Conversational competence and peer response to mildly retarded children. *Journal of Educational Psychology, 82,* 128–134.

Hubbell, R.D. (1988). *A handbook of English grammar and language sampling.* Englewood Cliffs, NJ: Prentice-Hall.

Hudson, J.A., & Shapiro, L.A. (1991). From knowledge to telling: The development of children's scripts, stories and person narratives. In C. Peterson & A. McCabe (Eds.), *Developing narrative structure* (pp. 89–136). Hillsdale, NJ: Lawrence Erlbaum Associates.

Ingram, D. (1972). The acquisition of the English verbal auxiliary and copula in normal and linguisically deviant children. *Papers and Reports on Child Language, 4,* 79–91.

Ito, T. (1986). Speech dysfluencies and acquisition of syntax in children 2–6 years old. *Folia Phoniatica, 38,* 310.

James, S.L. (1990). *Normal language acquisition.* Austin, TX: PRO-ED.

Janota, J. (1997). *American Speech-Language-Hearing Association Omnibus Survey* (ASHA Science and Research Department). Rockville, MD: American Speech-Language-Hearing Association.

Johnston, J.R. (1982). Narratives: A new look at communication problems in older language disordered children. *Language, Speech, and Hearing Services in Schools, 11,* 169–174.

Johnston, J.R. (1985). Fit, focus, and functionality: An essay in early language intervention. *Child Language Teaching and Therapy, 1,* 125–132.

Johnston, J.R. (1988) Specific language disorders in the child. In N. Lass, L. McReynolds, J. Northern, & D. Yoder

(Eds.), *Handbook of speech language pathology and audiology* (pp. 685–715). Philadelphia: B.C. Decker.

Johnston, J.R., & Kamhi, A.G. (1984). Syntactic and semantic aspects of the utterances of language-impaired children: The same can be less. *Merrill-Palmer Quarterly, 30,* 65–86.

Kail, R., & Leonard, L.B. (1986). *Word-finding abilities in language- impaired children.* ASHA Monographs #25. Rockville, MD: American Speech-Language-Hearing Association.

Kamhi, A. (1998). Trying to make sense of developmental language disorders. *Language, Speech, and Hearing Services in Schools, 29,* 35–44.

Kamhi, A., & Catts, H. (1989). *Reading disabilities: A developmental language perspective.* Boston: College-Hill Press.

Kamhi, A., & Johnston, J.J. (1982). Towards an understanding of retarded children's linguistic deficiencies. *Journal of Speech and Hearing Research, 25,* 435–445.

Kamhi, A., & Masterson, J. (1989). Language and cognition in mentally handicapped people: Last rites for the difference-delay controversy. In M. Beveridge, G. Conti-Ramsden, & I. Leuder (Eds.), *Language and communication in mentally handicapped people* (pp. 348–362). London: Chapman & Hall.

Kayser, H. (1989). Speech and language assessment of Spanish-English children. *Language, Speech, and Hearing Services in Schools, 20,* 226–241.

Kayser, H. (1995a). Bilingualism, myths, and language impairments. In H. Kayser (Ed.), *Bilingual speech-language pathology: An Hispanic focus* (pp. 185–206). San Diego: Singular Publication Group.

Kayser, H. (1995b). Intervention with children from linguistically and culturally diverse backgrounds. In M. Fey, J. Windsor, & S. Warren (Eds.), *Language intervention. Preschool through the elementary years* (pp. 315–332). Baltimore: Paul H. Brookes.

Kayser, H. (1998a). *Assessment and intervention resource for Hispanic children.* San Diego: Singular Publication Group.

Kayser, H. (1998b). Hispanic cultures and language. In. D. Battle (Ed.), *Communication disorders in multicultural populations* (pp. 157–196). Boston: Butterworth-Heinemann.

Kayser, H., & Restrepo, M.A. (1995). Language samples: Elicitation and analysis. In H. Kayser (Ed.), *Bilingual speech-language pathology: An Hispanic focus* (pp. 265–287). San Diego, CA: Singular Publication Group.

Kramer, C.A., James, S.L., & Saxman, J.H. (1979). A comparison of language samples elicited at home and in clinic. *Journal of Speech and Hearing Disorders, 44,* 321–330.

Labov, W. (1972). *Language in the inner city.* Philadelphia: University of Pennsylvania Press.

Lackner, J.R. (1968). A developmental study of language behavior in retarded children. *Neuropsychologia, 8,* 301–320.

Lahey, M. (1988). *Language disorders and language development.* New York: Macmillan.

Lahey, M. (1990). Who shall be called language disordered? Some reflections and one perspective. *Journal of Speech and Hearing Disorders, 55,* 612–620.

Langdon, H. (1992). Speech and language assessment of LEP/bilingual Hispanic students. In H. Langdon & L.R. Cheng (Eds.), *Hispanic children and adults with communication disorders* (pp. 201–271). Gaithersburg, MD: Aspen.

Larson, L.V., & McKinley, N. (1995). *Language disorders in older students: Preadolescents and adolescents.* Eau Claire, WI: Thinking Publications.

Leadholm, B., & Miller, J. (1992). *Language sample analysis: The Wisconsin guide.* Madison: Wisconsin Department of Public Instruction.

Leahy, R., Balla, D., & Zigler, E. (1982). Role-taking, self-image, and imitativeness of mentally retarded and nonretarded individuals. *American Journal of Mental Deficiency, 86,* 372–379.

Lee, L. (1966). Developmental sentence types: A method for comparing normal and deviant syntactic development. *Journal of Speech and Hearing Disorders, 31,* 311–330.

Lee, L. (1974). *Developmental sentence analysis.* Evanston, IL: Northwestern University Press.

Leonard, L.B. (1972). What is deviant language? *Journal of Speech and Hearing Disorders, 37,* 427–447.

Leonard, L.B. (1982). The nature of specific language impairment in children. In S. Rosenberg (Ed.), *Handbook of applied psycholinguistics* (pp. 295–328). Hillsdale, NJ: Erlbaum.

Leonard, L.B. (1991). Specific language impairment as a clinical category. *Language, Speech, Hearing Services in Schools, 22,* 66–68.

Leonard, L.B. (1995). Functional categories in the grammars of children with specific language impairment. *Journal of Speech and Hearing Research, 38,* 1270–1283.

Leonard, L.B. (1998). *Children with specific language impairment.* Cambridge, MA: The MIT Press.

Leonard, L.B., Bolders, J.G., & Miller, J.A. (1976). An examination of the semantic relations reflected in the language usage of normal and language-disordered children. *Journal of Speech and Hearing Research, 19,* 371–392.

Leonard, L.B., Camarata, S., Rowan, L.E., & Chapman, K. (1982). The communicative functions of lexical usage by language impaired children. *Applied Psycholinguistics, 3,* 109–125.

Leonard, L.B., Miller, C., & Gerber, E. (1999). Grammatical morphology and the lexicon of children with specific language impairment. *Journal of Speech, Language, and Hearing Research, 42,* 678–689.

Leonard, L.B., Nippold, M., Kail, R., & Hale, C. (1983). Picture naming in language-impaired children. *Journal of Speech and Hearing Research, 26,* 609–615.

Levitt, H., McGarr, N., & Geffner, D. (1987). Concluding commentary. In H. Levitt, N. McGarr, & D. Geffner (Eds.),

Development of language and communication skills in hearing-impaired children. *Asha Monographs, 26,* 140–145.

Liles, B.Z. (1993). Narrative discourse in children with language disorders and children with normal language: A critical review of the literature. *Journal of Speech and Hearing Research, 36,* 868–882.

Long, S.H. (1994). Language and children with autism. In V.A. Reed (Ed.), *An introduction to children with language disorders* (2nd ed.) (pp. 230–256). Boston: Allyn and Bacon.

Long, S.H., & Long, S.T. (1994). Language and children with learning disabilities. In V.A. Reed (Ed.) *An introduction to children with language disorders* (2nd ed.) (pp. 192–229). Boston: Allyn and Bacon.

Lucas, E.V. (1980). *Semantic and pragmatic language disorders.* Rockville, MD: Aspen.

Lund, N.J., & Duchan, J.F. (1993). *Assessing children's language in naturalistic contexts* (3rd ed.). Englewood Cliffs, NJ: Prentice-Hall.

MacLachlan, B., & Chapman, R. (1988). Communication breakdowns in normal and language learning-disabled children's conversation and narration. *Journal of Speech and Hearing Disorders, 53,* 2–7.

MacDonald, J. (1985). Language through conversation: A model for intervention with language-delayed persons. In S. Warren & A. Rogers-Warren (Eds.), *Teaching functional language: Generalization and maintenance of language skills* (pp. 89–122). Baltimore: University Park Press.

Mahoney, G.J. (1975). Ethological approach to delayed language acquisition. *American Journal of Mental Deficiency, 80,* 139–148.

Matheny, A.P. (1968). Pathological echoic responses in a child: Effect of environmental mand and tack control. *Journal of Experimental Child Psychology, 6,* 624–631.

McCabe, A., & Rollins, P.R. (1994). Assessment of preschool narrative skills. Prequisite for literacy. *American Journal of Speech-Language Pathology: A Journal of Clinical Practice, 13,* 45–56.

McGregor, K.K. (1997). The nature of word-finding errors of preschoolers with and without word-finding deficits. *Journal of Speech, Language, and Hearing Research, 40,* 1232–1244.

McGregor, K.K., & Leonard, L.B. (1989). Facilitating word-finding skills of language impaired children. *Journal of Speech and Hearing Disorders, 54,* 141–147.

McGregor, K.K., Williams, D., Hearst, S., & Johnson, S. (1997). The use of contrastive analysis in distinguishing difference from disorder: A tutorial. *American Journal of Speech-Language Pathology, 6,* 48–54.

McGregor, K.K., & Windsor, J. (1996). Effects of priming on the naming accuracy of preschoolers with word-finding difficulties. *Journal of Speech and Hearing Research, 39,* 1048–1058.

McKirdy, L., & Blank, M. (1982). Dialogue in deaf and hearing preschoolers. *Journal of Speech and Hearing Research, 25,* 487–499.

McLauglin, S. (1998). *Introduction to language development.* San Diego: Singular Publishing Group.

McShane, J. (1980). *Learning to talk.* Cambridge, MA: Cambridge University Press.

Mentis, M. (1994) Topic management in discourse: Assessment and intervention. *Topics in Language Disorders, 14,* 29–54.

Menyuk, P. (1964). Comparison of grammar of children with functionally deviant and normal speech. *Journal of Speech and Hearing Research, 7,* 109–121.

Menyuk, P. (1969). *Sentences children use.* Cambridge, MA: The MIT Press.

Menyuk, P. (1977). *Language and maturation.* Cambridge, MA: The MIT Press.

Miranda, A.E., McCabe, A., & Bliss, L.S. (1998). Jumping around and leaving things out: A profile of the narrative abilities of children with specific language impairment. *Applied Psycholinguistics, 19,* 647–667.

Montgomery, J.K. (1999). Accents and dialects: Creating a national professional statement. *Topics in Language Disorders, 19,* 78–86.

Morehead, D.M., & Ingram, D. (1973). The development of base syntax in normal and linguistically deviant children. *Journal of Speech and Hearing Research, 16,* 330–353.

Naremore, R.C., Densmore, A.E., & Harman, D.R. (1995). *Language intervention with school-aged children.* San Diego: Singular Publishing Group.

Nelson, K.E., Camarata, S.M., Welsh, J., Butkovsky, L., & Camarata, M. (1996). Effects of imitative and conversational recasting treatment on the acquisition of grammar in children with specific language impairment and younger language-normal children. *Journal of Speech and Hearing Research, 39,* 850–859.

Nelson, N.W. (1988). *Planning individualized speech and language intervention programs* (2nd ed.). Tucson, AZ: Communication Skill Builders.

Nelson, N.W. (1998). *Childhood language disorders in context. Infancy through adolescence* (2nd ed.). Boston: Allyn and Bacon.

Nelson, N.W., & Hyter, Y.D. (1990). How to use Black English sentence scoring (BESS) as a tool of non-biased assessment. Short course presented at the American Speech-Language-Hearing Association convention, Seattle, WA.

Nippold, M.A. (1988). Introduction. In M.A. Nippold (Ed.), *Later language development* (pp. 1–10). San Diego: College-Hill Press.

Nippold, M.A. (1993). Developmental markers in adolescent language: Syntax, semantics and pragmatics. *Language, Speech and Hearing Services in Schools, 24,* 21–28.

Nippold, M.A. (2000). Language development during the adolescent years: Aspects of pragmatics, syntax and semantics. *Topics in Language Disorders, 20,* 15–28.

Norris, J.A., & Hoffman, P.R. (1993). *Whole language intervention for school aged children.* San Diego: Singular Publishing Group.

Northern, J.L., & Downs, M.P. (1984). *Hearing in children* (3rd ed.), Baltimore: Williams & Wilkins.

Oetting, J.B., & Rice, M.L. (1991). Influence of the social context on pragmatic skills of adults with mental retardation. *American Journal of Mental Retardation, 95,* 435–443.

Olswang, L.B., & Carpenter, R.L. (1978). Elicitor effects on the language obtained from young language impaired children. *Journal of Speech and Hearing Disorders, 43,* 76–88.

Owens, R.E. (1996). *Language development: An introduction* (4th ed.). Boston: Allyn and Bacon.

Owens, R.E. (1997). Mental retardation: Difference and delay. In D.K. Bernstein and E. Tiegerman-Farber (Eds.), *Language and communication disorders in children* (4th ed.) (pp. 457–523). Boston: Allyn and Bacon.

Owens, R.E. (1999). *Language disorders. A functional approach to assessment and intervention* (3rd ed.). Boston: Allyn and Bacon.

Owens, R.E., & MacDonald, J.D. (1982). Communicative uses of the early speech of nondelayed and Down Syndrome children. *American Journal of Mental Deficiency, 86,* 503–510.

Paccia Cooper, J., & Curcio, F. (1970). Language processing and forms of echolalia in severely disturbed children. Unpublished manuscript.

Paul, R. (1981). Complex sentence development. In J. Miller (Ed.), *Assessing language production in children* (pp. 69–71). Baltimore: University Park Press.

Paul, R. (2001). *Childhood language disorders in context. Infancy through adolescence.* (2nd ed.). Boston: Allyn and Bacon.

Pearson, B.Z., Fernández, S.C., & Oller, D.K. (1993). Lexical development in bilingual infants and toddlers: Comparison to monolingual norms. *Language Learning, 43,* 93–120.

Peña, E.D., & Jackson, J.E. (2000). The social and cultural bases of communication. In R.B. Gillam, P. Marquardt, & F.N. Martin (Eds.), *Communication sciences and disorders. From science to clinical practice.* San Diego: Singular Publishing Group, Thomson Learning.

Peterson, C., & McCabe, A. (1983). *Developmental psycholinguistics: Three ways of looking at a child's narrative.* New York: Plenum.

Piaget, J. (1926). *The language and thought of the child.* London: Routledge & Keagan Paul.

Prizant, B.M. (1982). Gestalt language and gestalt processing in autism. *Topics in Language Disorders, 3,* 16–24.

Prizant, B.M., & Duchan, J.F. (1981). The functions of immediate echolalia in autistic children. *Journal of Speech and Hearing Disorders, 46,* 241–249.

Prizant, B.M., & Rydell, P.J. (1984). Analysis of functions of delayed echolalia in autistic children. *Journal of Speech and Hearing Research, 27,* 183–192.

Purcell, S.L., & Liles, B.Z. (1992). Cohesion repairs in the narratives of normal-language and language disordered school aged children. *Journal of Speech and Hearing Research, 35,* 354–362.

Quigley, S. (1978). Effects of hearing impairment on normal language development. In F. Martin (Ed.), *Pediatric audiology.* Englewood Cliffs, NJ: Prentice-Hall.

Quigley, S., & Paul, P.V. (1984). *Language and deafness.* Austin, TX: PRO-ED.

Quigley, S., Power, D.J., & Stenkamp, M.W. (1977). The language structure of deaf children. *The Volta Review, 79,* 73–84.

Quigley, S. Smith, N., & Wilbur, R. (1974). Comprehension of relativized sentences by deaf students. *Journal of Speech and Hearing Research, 17,* 325–341.

Radziewicz, D., & Antonellis, S. (1997). Considerations and implications for habilitation of hearing impaired children. In D.K Bernstein & E. Tiegerman-Farber (Ed.), *Language and communication disorders in children* (pp. 574–603). Boston: Allyn and Bacon.

Records, N.L., Tomblin, J.B., & Freese, P.R. (1992). Quality of life in adults with histories of specific language impairment. *American Journal of Speech-Language Pathology, 1,* 44–53.

Reed, V.A. (1994). Assessment and Diagnosis. In V.A. Reed (Ed.), *An introduction to children with language disorders* (pp. 416–441). New York: Merrill/Macmillan.

Restrepo, M.A. (1998). Identifiers of predominantly Spanish-speaking children with language impairment. *Journal of Speech, Language, and Hearing Research, 41,* 1398–1411.

Retherford, K.S. (1993). *Guide to analysis of language transcripts* (2nd ed.). Eau Claire, WI: Thinking Publications.

Retherford, K.S., Schwartz, R.C., & Chapman, R.S. (1981). Semantic roles and residual grammatical categories in mother and child speech: Who tunes into whom? *Journal of Child Language, 8,* 563–608.

Rice, M.L. (1994). Grammatical categories of children with specific language impairments. In R.V. Watkins & M.L. Riche (Eds.), *Specific language impairments in children* (pp. 69–89). Baltimore: Paul H. Brookes.

Rice, M. L., & Oetting, J.A. (1993). Morphological deficits of children with specific language impairment: Evaluation of number marking and agreement. *Journal of Speech and Hearing Research, 36,* 1249–1257.

Rice, M.L., & Wexler, K. (1996). Toward tense as a clinical marker of specific language impairment in English-Speaking children. *Journal of Speech and Hearing Research, 39,* 1239–1257.

Rom, A., & Bliss, L.S. (1981). A comparison of verbal communicative skills of language-impaired and normal-speaking children. *Journal of Communicative Disorders, 14,* 133–140.

Rosenberg, S. (1982). The language of the mentally retarded: Development, processes and intervention. In S. Rosenberg (Ed.), *Handbook of applied psycholinguistics* (pp. 329–392). Hillsdale, NJ: Lawrence Erlbaum.

Rosenthal, W., Eisenson, J., & Luckau, J. (1972). A statistical test of the validity of the diagnostic categories used in childhood language disorders: Implications for assessment procedures. *Papers and Reports in Child Language Development, 4,* 121–143, Stanford University, Palo Alto, CA.

Russell, W.K., Quigley, S., & Power, D. J. (1976). *Linguistics and deaf children.* Washington, DC: The A.G. Bell Association for the Deaf.

Rutter, M. (1968). Concepts of autism: A review of research. *Journal of Child Psychology, 9,* 1–25.

Sachs, J., & Devin, J. (1976). Young children's use of age appropriate speech styles. *Journal of Child Language, 15,* 381–98.

Schuler, A.L. (1979). Echolalia: Issues and clinical applications. *Journal of Speech and Hearing Disorders, 44,* 411–434.

Scott, C.S. (1988). Spoken and written syntax. In M.A. Nippold (Ed.), *Later language development* (pp. 49–96). San Diego: College-Hill Press.

Scott, C.S. (1994). A discourse continuum for school-age students: Impact of modality and genre. In G.P. Wallach and K.G. Butler (Eds.), *Language learning disabilities in school-age children and adolescents* (pp. 219–252). New York: Merrill.

Scott, C.M., & Stokes, S.L. (1995). Measures of syntax in school-age children and adolescents. *Language, Speech, and Hearing Services in Schools, 26,* 309–317.

Scott, C.M., & Windsor, J. (2000). General language performance measures in spoken and written narrative and expository discourse of school age children with language learning disabilities. *Journal of Speech, Language, and Hearing Research, 43,* 324–339.

Seidenberg, P.L. (1997). Understanding learning disabilities. In D.K. Bernstein & E. Tiegerman-Farber (Eds.), *Language and communication disorders in children* (4th ed.) (pp. 413–456). Boston: Allyn and Bacon.

Seymour, H.N., Abdulkarim, L., & Johnson, V. (1999). The Ebonics controversy: An educational and clinical dilemma. *Topics in Language Disorders, 19,* 66–71.

Seymour, H.N., Bland-Stewart, L., & Green, L.J. (1998). Difference versus deficit in child African American English. *Language, Speech, and Hearing Services in Schools, 29,* 96–108.

Seymour, H.N., & Roeper, T. (1999). Grammatical acquisiton of African American English. In O. Taylor and L.B. Leonard (Eds.), *Language acquisiton across north America* (pp. 109–154). San Diego: Singular Publishing Group.

Shantz, C.U. (1983). The role of role-taking in children's referential communication. In W.P. Dickson (Ed.), *Children's oral communication skills* (pp. 85–102). New York: Academic Press.

Shatz, M., & Gelman, R. (1973). The development of communication skills: Modifications in the speech of young children as a function of the listener. *Monographs of the Society for Research in Child Development, 38* (Serial No. 152).

Shaw, S.D. (1994). Language and hearing-impaired children. In V. Reed (Ed.), *An introduction to children with language disorders* (pp. 257–289). Boston: Allyn and Bacon.

Silva, M.J., & McCabe, A. (1996). Vignettes of the continuous and family ties: Some Latino American traditions. In A. McCabe (Ed.) *Chameleon readers: Teaching children to appreciate all kinds of good stories* (pp. 116–136). New York: McGraw-Hill.

Singer, B.D., & Bashir, A.S. (1999). What are executive functions and self-regulation and what do they have to do with language-learning disorders? *Language, Speech, and Hearing Services in Schools, 30,* 265–273.

Skarakis, E., & Prutting, C. A. (1977). Early communication: Semantic functions and communicative intentions in the communication of the preschool child with impaired hearing. *American Annals of the Deaf, 122,* 383–391.

Smitherman, G.S. (1977). *Talkin' and testifyin'.* Boston: Houghton Mifflin.

Smitherman, G.S. (1983). This Black language thang. Linguistic characteristics of Black English. In L. Bliss & D.V. Allen, *Screening Kit of Language Development.* Aurora, NY: Slosson.

Sonnenschien, S. (1986). Development of referential communication skills: How familiarity with a listener affects a speaker's production of redundant messages. *Developmental Psychology, 22,* 549–552.

Steffani, S., & Olson, L.S. (1998). Identifying complex sentences: Making it simple. Presentation at the American Speech-Language-Hearing Association Convention, San Antonio, TX.

Stinson, M.S., & Whitmire, K.A. (2000). Adolescents who are deaf or hard of hearing: A communicative perspective on educational placement. *Topics in Language Disorders, 20,* 58–72.

Stockman, I.J. (1996). The promises and pitfalls of language sample analysis as an assessment tool for linguistic minority children. *Language, Speech, and Hearing Services in Schools, 27,* 355–366.

Strothard, S.E., Snowling, M.V., Bishop, D.W.M., Chipchase, B.B., & Kaplan, C.A. (1998). Language impaired preschoolers: A follow-up into adolescence. *Journal of Speech, Language, and Hearing Research, 41,* 407–415.

Tager-Flusberg, H., & Calkins, S. (1990). Does imitation facilitate the acquisition of grammar? Evidence from a study of autistic, Down's syndrome and normal children. *Journal of Child Language, 17,* 591–606.

Taylor, O.L. (1985). *Nature of communication disorders in culturally and linguistically diverse populations.* Austin, TX: PRO-ED.

Terrell, S.L., Battle, D.E., & Granthan, R.B. (1998). *Communication disorders in multicultural populations* (2nd ed.) (pp. 31–72). Boston: Butterworth-Heinemann.

Terrell, S.L., & Terrell, F. (1993). African-American cultures. In D.E. Battle (Ed.), *Communication disorders in multicultural populations* (pp. 3–37). Stoneham, MA: Butterworth-Heinemann.

Tiegerman-Farber, E. (1997). Autism: Learning to communicate. In D.K. Bernstein and E. Tiegerman-Farber (Eds.), *Language and communication disorders in children* (4th ed.) (pp. 524–573). Boston: Allyn and Bacon.

Tomblin, J.B., Records, N.L., Buckwalter, P., Zhang, X., Smith, E., & O'Brien, M. (1997). Prevalence of SLI in kindergarten children. *Journal of Speech and Hearing Research, 40*, 1245–1260.

Tomblin, J.B., Records, N.L., & Zhang, X. (1996). A system for the diagnosis of specific language impairment in kindergarten children. *Journal of Speech and Hearing Research, 39*, 1284–1294.

Turkstra, L.S., & Holland, A.L. (1998). Assessment of syntax after adolescent brain injury: Effects of memory on test performance. *Journal of Speech and Hearing Research, 41*, 137–149.

U.S. Bureau of the Census (1996). *Statistical abstract of the United States: 1996* (116th ed.). Washington, DC: U.S. Bureau of the Census.

Van Keulen, J.E., Weddington, G.T., & DeBose, C.E. (1998). *Speech, language, learning and the African American child.* Boston: Allyn and Bacon.

Vaughn-Cooke, F.B. (1983). Improving language assessment in minority children. *Asha, 25*, 29–34.

Violette, J., & Swisher, L. (1992). Echolalic responses by a child with autism to four experimental conditions of sociolinguistic input. *Journal of Speech and Hearing Research, 35*, 139–147.

Vygotsky, L.S. (1962). *Thought and language* (edited and translated by E. Hanfmann & G. Vakar from the original work, published posthumously in 1934). Cambridge, MA: MIT Press.

Wagner, C.R., Nettelbladtt, U., Sahlen, B., & Nilholm, C. (2000). Conversation versus narration in preschool children with language impairment. *International Journal of Language and Communication Disorders, 35*, 83–93.

Washington, J.A. (1996). Issues in assessing the language abilities of African American children. In A.G. Kamhi, K.E. Pollock, & J.L. Harris (Eds.), *Communication development and disorders in African American children* (pp. 35–54). Baltimore: Paul H. Brookes.

Washington, J., & Craig, H. (1992). Performances of low-income, African American preschool and kindergarten children on the Peabody Picture Vocabulary Test—Revised. *Language, Speech, and Hearing Services in Schools, 23*, 329–333.

Washington, J.A., & Craig, H. (1994). Dialectal forms during discourse of urban African American preschoolers living in poverty. *Journal of Speech and Hearing Research, 37*, 816–823.

Washington, J.A., Craig, H.K., & Kushman, A.J. (1998). Variable use of African American English across two language sampling contexts. *Journal of Speech, Language, and Hearing Research, 41*, 1115–1124.

Watkins, R.V. (1994). Grammatical challenges for children with specific language impairments. In R.V. Watkins and M.L. Rice (Eds.), *Specific language impairments in children* (pp. 53–68). Baltimore: Paul H. Brookes.

Weiss, A. (1986). Classroom discourse and the hearing-impaired child. *Topics in Language Disorders, 6*, 60–70.

Wells, G. (1985). *Language development in the preschool years.* New York: Cambridge University.

Wetherby, A.M., Cain, D.H., Yonclas, D.G., & Walker, C.K. (1988). Analysis of intentional communication of normal children from the prelinguistic to the multiword stage. *Journal of Speech and Hearing Research, 31*, 240–252.

Wetherby, A.M., & Prutting, C.A. (1984). Profiles of communicative and cognitive-social abilities in autistic children. *Journal of Speech and Hearing Research, 27*, 364–377.

Whitmire, K.A. (2000). Adolescence as a developmental phase: A tutorial. *Topics in Language Disorders, 20*, 1–14.

Wiig, E.H. (1995). Assessment of adolescent language. *Seminars in Speech and Language, 16*, 14–31.

Wiig, E.H., & Semel, E.M., (1984). *Language assessment and intervention for the learning disabled.* Columbus, OH: Merrill.

Wolfram, W. (1986). Language variation in the United States. In O. Taylor (Ed.), *Nature of communication disorders in culturally and linguistically diverse populations* (pp. 128–157). San Diego: College-Hill Press.

Wyatt, T. (1997). The Oakland Ebonics debate: Implications for speech, language, hearing professionals and scholars. *Special Interest Division One Newsletter: Language Learning and Education, 4*, 15–18.

Wyatt, T.A. (1996). Acquisition of the African American English copula. In A.G. Kamhi, K.E. Pollock, & J.L. Harris (Eds.), *Communication development and disorders in African American children* (pp. 95–116). Baltimore: Paul H. Brookes.

Ylvisaker, M. (1992). Communication outcome following TBI. *Seminars in Speech and Language, 13*, 239–251.

Ylvisaker, M., & DuBonis, D. (2000). Executive function impairment in adolescence: TBI and ADHD, *Topics in Language Disorders, 20*, 29–57.

Ylvisaker, M., & Feeney, T.J. (1995). TBI in adolescence: Assessment and reintegration. *Seminars in Speech and Language, 16*, 32–45.

Ylvisaker, M., & Szekeres, S.F. (1989). Metacognitive and executive impairments in head-injured children and adults. *Topics in Language Disorders, 9*, 34–49.

Yoshinaga-Itano, C. (1986). Beyond the sentence level: What's in a hearing impaired child's story? *Topics in Language Disorders, 6*, 71–83.

Index